REFLECTIVE PRACTICE
FOR NURSES

Student Survival Skills Series

Survive your nursing course with these essential guides for all student nurses:

Medicine Management Skills for Nurses, 2nd Edition
Claire Boyd
9781119807926

Clinical Skills for Nurses, 2nd Edition
Claire Boyd
9781119871545

Study Skills for Nurses
Claire Boyd
9781118657430

Care Skills for Nurses
Claire Boyd
9781118657386

Communication Skills for Nurses
Claire Boyd and Janet Dare
9781118767528

Acute Care for Nurses
Claire Boyd
9781119882459

Calculation Skills for Nurses, 2nd Edition
Claire Boyd
9781119808121

Wellbeing Strategies for Nurses
Claire Boyd
9781119893554

REFLECTIVE PRACTICE
FOR NURSES

Claire Boyd
RGN, Cert Ed
Practice Development Trainer

WILEY Blackwell

Registered Offices
John Wiley & Sons, Inc., 111 River Street, Hoboken, NJ 07030, USA
John Wiley & Sons Ltd, The Atrium, Southern Gate, Chichester, West Sussex, PO19 8SQ, UK

For details of our global editorial offices, customer services, and more information about Wiley products visit us at www.wiley.com.

Wiley also publishes its books in a variety of electronic formats and by print-on-demand. Some content that appears in standard print versions of this book may not be available in other formats.

Library of Congress Cataloging-in-Publication Data Applied for

Paperback: 9781119882480

Cover Design: Wiley
Cover Images: © rambo182/Getty Images

Set in 9/12pt Trade Gothic Light by Straive, Pondicherry, India
Printed and bound by CPI Group (UK) Ltd, Croydon CR0 4YY
C9781119882480_211222

Contents

CONTENTS

Preface

Reflective Practice for Nurses is part of a series of books for the student nurse. The books are, however, designed for any healthcare professional requiring a little assistance in the topic matter – in this case, nursing reflection.

The whole book series is designed to be easy to read, with short, snappy explanations.

As with other books in this series, the book has been divided into three sections:

Section One – 'Understanding Reflection', where we will look at 14 models of reflection.

Section Two – 'Learning through Reflection', where we will look at how reflection can improve our care

Section Three – 'Reflection in Practice', where we will look at some real-life case studies and a reflective journal extract

Each chapter is laid out in a simple-to-follow, step-by-step approach and ends with a 'Test Your Knowledge' section to assist your understanding. The aim of the book is to start you on a journey of using reflection in your practice, from day one to qualification and beyond. It has been compiled using quotes and tips from student nurses themselves.

Introduction

I began my nursing career at the age of four. I had a ward full of patients to care for: unfortunately, despite my best efforts, Panda did not make it.

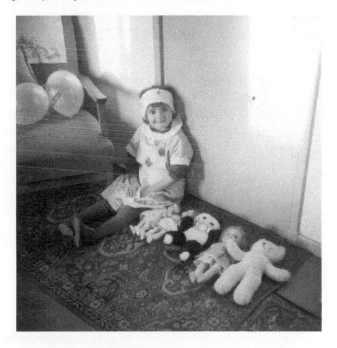

My elder brother came into my ward and stole away one of my patients. I had three options:

1   Cry and call out for 'Mummy'!!
2   Calmly talk to the kidnapper, discussing the error of his ways
3   Run after my brother, and bite him as hard as I could

With hindsight, option 3, the option I went for, was probably not the best choice!

More recently, sitting at my brother's bedside as he approached his end of life, we laughed at this childhood incident and the bite scar on his stomach, which he carried for the rest of his life.

As I grew up, my nursing career continued, starting off by working for a nursing agency as a nursing auxilliary, which fitted in well with my family and fostering children. I then undertook my training at the University of the West of England to become a registered general nurse, followed by undertaking a certificate in education to teach those in the nursing profession. I have now been a nurse and practice development trainer for 40 years.

Throughout my career, I have made mistakes, but learning from these mistakes has made me a better nurse. Reflection has been an important part in this process. As a student nurse/midwife, you will also gain an understanding of this reflection process; choosing the correct model of reflection to use will be an important step in this direction.

An important element to our professional development for our Nursing and Midwifery Council (NMC) is revalidation, which includes five written reflective accounts. We will look into this and the other NMC requirements of revalidation in Chapter 4.

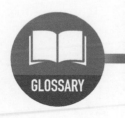

GLOSSARY

Revalidation

This is the mechanism used to confirm or establish the continuing competence of health practitioners by proving that their skills are up-to-date and that they remain fit to practice. The intention of revalidation is to reassure patients, employers, and other professionals and to improve patient care and safety.

If this all seems a little daunting, don't worry: this book will guide you through the reflective practice in nursing, showing real-life case studies and how reflective practice can assist you by allowing you to identify areas for learning and development and how you can put changes or improvements into action in your everyday practice as a result. This book includes hints and tips from healthcare professionals just like you, helping you to make sense of reflective practice in nursing.

Perhaps as a nursing student this will be your first foray into the world of reflection (and you may have even wondered why we have information on revalidation): I can assure you, it will be no time at all until you qualify and will therefore have a heads-up of the process of reflection and revalidation.

Reflection is a life-long process whereby you will learn the foundations of the process before applying it to practice; this book aims to give you these building blocks.

Lastly, there are boxes titled 'Student Tips', 'Glossary', 'Did You Know?' and 'Web Resources', with a dash of humour, as I fully understand that textbooks can be a bit heavy sometimes and there is nothing wrong with a quick change of pace!

DID YOU KNOW?

I went to casualty yesterday and said to the nurse, 'I've been stung by a wasp! Have you got anything for it?'
Nurse asked, 'Whereabouts is it?'
I said, 'I don't know, it could be miles away by now!' LOL.

—Claire Boyd
Bristol

WEB RESOURCES

Reflection: https://www.nursingtimes.net/roles/
nurse-educators/a-new-model-of-reflection-for-clinical-practice-17-08-2015/
NMC Code of Conduct: https://www.nmc.org.uk/standards/code/
This site will also direct you to online revalidation forms and templates:

- Practice hours log template
- CPD log template
- Feedback log template
- Reflective accounts form
- Reflective discussion form
- Confirmation form
- Combined revalidation forms and templates
- Completed forms and templates
- 'Support to help you revalidate' guidance sheet

Acknowledgements

Acknowledgements go first and foremost to the student nurses from the University of the West of England (UWE) and others from North Bristol NHS Trust who contributed to the contents of this book. Your reflections are, as promised, confidential adaptations and anonymous.

Thanks also go to all those behind-the-scenes professionals at Blackwell's Wiley – Tom Marriott (commissioning editor), Ella Elliott (editorial assistant), Tiffany Taylor (copyeditor), Sathishwaran (Content Refinement Specialist) Anne Hunt (publishing assistant), and everyone else at Blackwell's: thank you all for helping me to develop this series of books, which I know through feedback from the readers have helped in their studies and/or professional development.

Lastly, thanks go to my family (husband Rob and son Simon) for supplying food and cups of coffee when I had my head deep in research notes and interview tapes and knowing when to 'leave me to it'. Thanks also to Louise and David, and grandsons Owen and Rhys, who I never minded disturbing me and making Granny laugh! Loved your joke, Owen, about 'What is black and white, black and white, black and white? A penguin rolling down a hill!' What made me laugh more was seeing how both you and Rhys laughed hysterically at the joke – and baby Rhys didn't even understand the joke! Never lose your sense of humour, boys, no matter what life throws at you.

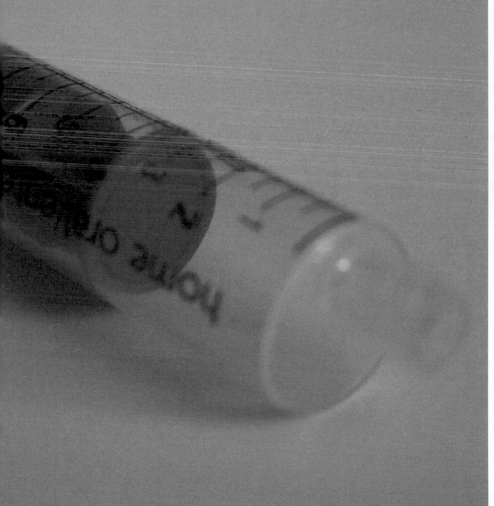

Section One
· · · · · · · · · · · · · · · · · · · ·
UNDERSTANDING REFLECTION

Chapter 1

. . . .

WHAT IS REFLECTION?

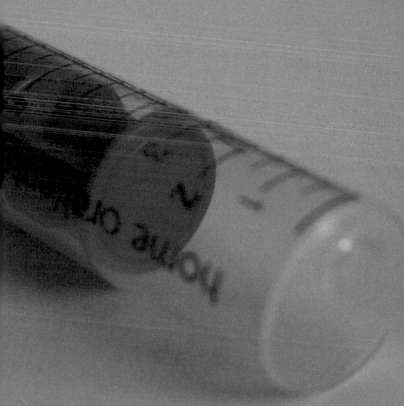

Reflective Practice for Nurses, First Edition. Claire Boyd.
© 2023 John Wiley & Sons Ltd. Published 2023 by John Wiley & Sons Ltd.

LEARNING OUTCOMES

By the end of this chapter, you should have a working knowledge of the different types of reflection and how the process of reflection can enhance our nursing practice and learning.

Training in healthcare, you will find the skill of using reflection deeply embedded in the learning process of nurse education and practice.

When I began my nursing career (no, not alongside the pioneers of nursing, Mary Seacole and Florence Nightingale – cheeky!), the concept of 'reflection' as a learning aid was still considered quite new and in its infancy. I can remember some of my colleagues stating that reflection was 'a flash in the pan' and would be replaced by the 'next new thing': it was obvious that they had not yet fully understood the value and importance of reflection as an aid to enhance their learning and their nursing practice.

Reflection has been used in nursing and midwifery for many decades in many different guises – nurses with many years of experience under their belts all remember the SWOT (Strength, Weakness, Opportunities, Threats) analysis, still used today in many appraisals (we will look at a SWOT analysis and appraisals in Chapter 4). Reflection is also a process that we all engage in naturally to some extent; we may encounter a patient and wonder to ourselves, 'Why did he respond that way to me?'

Today, reflection in nursing and many other professions (such as teaching) is recognised for its benefits in helping us to learn and in professional development.

DID YOU KNOW?

Reflection is not just to do with the subject matter of **what** we are thinking about or learning but **how** we think about it and how we learn.

As a student nurse/midwife, and even after we have qualified in the nursing profession, we may be asked to produce the following, all containing one or more elements of **reflection**:

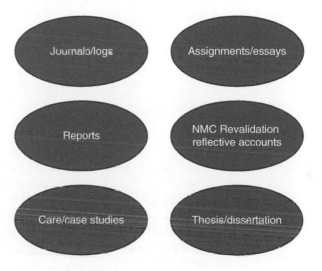

Journals/logs

Assignments/essays

Reports

NMC Revalidation reflective accounts

Care/case studies

Thesis/dissertation

DEFINITION OF REFLECTION

So what exactly is reflection? A definition of 'reflection' may mean different things to different people, but it can be said to describe learning from experience or even thinking with a purpose.

Today, nurses engaging in the revalidation process (which we will explore in Chapter 3) understand how the reflective practice can be an aid in learning and promoting good practice.

Research (Clarke 2014) tells us that there are 10 essential ingredients for successful reflection:

1 Academic skills
2 Knowledge
3 Attitudinal qualities
4 Self-awareness
5 Being person-centred

6 Being empathic
7 Communication
8 Mindfulness
9 Being process-orientated
10 Being strategic

TYPES OF REFLECTION

Reflection may be said to be informal or formal.

Informal Reflection

This provides recognition that learning has taken place. It could take the form of spending a little time at the end of each day to write in a log and consider what you have learned, identifying further learning you want to undertake, or considering how you want to understand or think about how you may improve your practice. **No one else ever needs to see this personal account unless you wish to share it with someone you trust to gain another perspective.**

As informal learning may be unstructured, it may be a good idea to bring some structure to the process. This is often achieved by asking yourself

- What went well today?
- What did not go so well?
- What would you do differently next time?

Informal learning is a valuable learning aid even if it often results in superficial learning. More meaningful reflection and learning can be undertaken by the formal approach to reflection.

Formal Reflection

Formal reflection may be used during the capability process, perhaps after making a mistake in the workplace, to establish your learning from this mistake. Examples of these can be seen in Chapters 9–14.

Formal reflection is also the approach we need to undertake during revalidation (Chapter 4): as part of the revalidation process (every three years), it is mandatory that we produce five reflective accounts and demonstrate that we have learned from events. **These reflections will be seen by and discussed with your confirmer** so that we are able to develop our practice. The Nursing and Midwifery Council (NMC) reflective account must be based on one or more of the following:

- An instance of your continuing professional development (CPD)
- A piece of practice-related feedback you have received
- An event or experience in your own professional practice and how this relates to the code

We will look at the process of revalidation more closely in Chapter 4, but it should be understood that revalidation only applies once you have qualified.

The five pieces of reflection can contain what is good about your practice. Following is a reflective piece used in my own revalidation some time ago; it concerns receiving feedback (praise) from a group of first-year student nurses who attended a calculations master class I was delivering.

Reflective Account: Calculations Master Class (Evaluation Form Feedback)

What was the nature of the CPD activity and/or practice-related feedback and/or event or experience in your practice?

I delivered a Calculations Master Class to year 1 student nurses and am aware that mathematics is often a problem to participants with a 'fear of maths' for many individuals. I therefore try to add humour to diffuse the teaching sessions in order to relax them and aid their learning.

What did you learn from the CPD activity and/or feedback and/or event or experience in your practice?

Good to know that some of these nervous learners found my training event to be 'useful' and in some instances, even 'enjoyable'. I will therefore continue to incorporate this technique to all my teaching sessions, where appropriate. I will however need to be mindful when using humour as humour is very subjective.

How did you change or improve your practice as a result?

I read articles, during my Certificate of Education course, about using humour in the learning environment, and how beneficial this can be, especially in topics not best liked by Participants i.e. calculations.

How is this relevant to the Code?

- *Practice effectively – 6, 7, 8, and 9*
- *Always practise in line with the best available evidence – 6*
- *Communicate clearly – 7*
- *Work co-operatively – 8*
- *Share your skills, knowledge and experience for the benefit of people receiving care and your colleagues - 9*

To be quite honest, this was a poor attempt, as it was far too brief and needed more 'meat on the bones' – in other words, it required much more information. Gibbs (1988) stated that 'It is not sufficient to have an experience in order to learn. Without reflecting on this experience, it may quickly be forgotten, or its learning potential lost'. Very little learning has taken place in the previous example, so I discarded this account and wrote a more-in-depth piece – but you can see the beginnings of reflective writing.

GIVING PRAISE

Did you notice how the earlier reflection concerned 'praise'? We will now look at a Nursing Associate's first attempt to use the reflective process without the structure of a nursing model:

I had a difficult shift and was very late going home. On my way down to the hospital lobby, I saw a newly qualified nurse I knew, and she was crying. When I went up to her to ask what the matter was, she told me that she had 'had the shift from hell'. We went to a quiet corner, out of the way, and I listened to the nurse's account. I was able to steer the conversation to finding resolutions to the issues that she raised. I was careful not to give my opinions, but let her come to her own conclusions. By the end of the discussion, she had stopped crying and even laughed about the situation.

Next shift, I received a 'thank you' card from this nurse, which made my day. It said how kind and empathetic I had been and what a lovely, caring nurse I am. I realised what receiving positive feedback means to individuals and how much difference this can make to people. Everyone loves praise, and I make sure I use positive praise in my daily working life and can see the impact of this on the morale of a team.

This is an excellent start in using the reflective process, but it would have been enhanced by using evidence to back up the claims that 'everyone loves praise'. This Nursing Associate could have stated, 'Research has shown that the power of praise creates a positive response that extends to enhancing the feeling of competence, improved motor skills performance, and increased motivation' and then cited this piece of evidence.

DID YOU KNOW?

'There are two things people want more than sex and money: Recognition and Praise.'

—Mary Kay Ash,
founder of Mary Kay Cosmetics

REFLECTIVE TERMINOLOGY

Beginning your journey into the world of reflection, you will no doubt hear many similar-sounding terms. This can lead to confusion. To aid your understanding, some of the terminology related to reflection can be seen in Table 1.1.

Table 1.1 Reflective terminology.

Term	Meaning
Reflection	Thinking with a purpose
Reflective practitioner	Healthcare professional who uses what they have learnt from experience to develop their knowledge and deliver the best care possible
Reflective practice	Thinking about a situation or experience and learning from it
Reflective processes	Structured methods/models that enable new actions to be based on learning gained from experience
Reflexive (or reflective)	Purposefully thoughtful; mindful
Writing reflectively	The process of writing a reflection
Reflective discussion	The process of talking with another person about a verbal or written reflection
Reflexivity	Using experiences to learn more about yourself
Critical reflection	Looking back on claims or assumptions and exploring, examining, and critiquing them
Reflection-on-practice	Looking back on an experience and learning from it
Reflection-in-practice	Reflection that happens while you are practicing, such as in an emergency situation
Anticipatory reflection	Action planning before an event occurs

WHY DO WE NEED TO REFLECT IN NURSING?

In short, to enhance our practice and our own professional development. In the nursing profession, we need to reflect due to

- **Professional body requirements**
  The NMC requires all nurses and midwives to maintain and develop their practice throughout their career.

- **Knowledge and Skills Framework (KSF)**
  This framework is applied in your practice and followed up in development reviews and personal development plans.
- **Course requirements**
  Healthcare professional training includes assignments and case studies that are reflective in nature, whereby theory is applied to practice, thereby beginning the process of becoming a healthcare lifelong learner.
- **Self-development**
  Reflection in practice is aimed at enhancing professional practice.

DID YOU KNOW?

Knowledge and Skills Framework (KSF): The NHS KSF was developed as part of the Agenda for Change (AfC) process for updating the way NHS staff posts are defined and developed.

The KSF defines and describes the knowledge and skills NHS staff need to apply in their work in order to deliver quality services.

WHY DO WE USE REFLECTION IN NURSING?

Reflection benefits not just the individual but also the patient and the organisation; see Figure 1.1.

The Reflective Process

We will look at tools, frameworks, or models (whatever you want to call them!) of reflection in Chapter 4, but we can

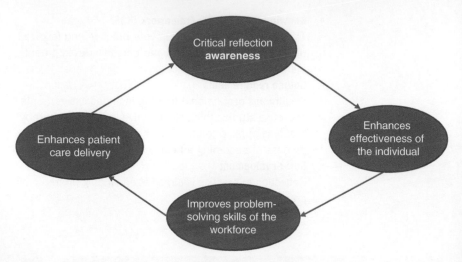

Figure 1.1 Some of the benefits of reflection.

start with the premise that the act of reflection, in a professional sense, should contain these six essential elements:

- Incident/experience (positive or negative)
- A description
- An analysis
- An interpretation
- A perspective
- An action

In short, it is no good reflecting about an incident or experience without taking some learning from it. At a basic level, this is what comes to my mind when using reflection in my nursing practice:

This is what happened
How do I feel?
Could I have done anything differently?
Planning a course of action (analysing and exploration)
What I have learnt – acquiring knowledge and skills (life-long)

As you can see, reflection does not have to be some convoluted, high-brow process; this is why it is important to find a reflective model that works for you. Personally, I would never use Kolb's experiential learning cycle (Chapter 4) as I find it too complex with its words like 'conceptualisation'. Some of my colleagues do like to use this model of reflection – to each their own!

BEGINNING OUR ENGAGEMENT WITH THE REFLECTIVE PROCESS

Johns, who has written much about the reflective process, suggests that we can begin our engagement with the reflective process by

- Being open to learning about ourselves
- Being able to acknowledge what our attitudes and perceptions are
- Being open and challenging our current ideologies
- Having the ability to be empathic
- Being able to view the world as others may see it
- Being able to combine evidence-based theory with our 'personal knowing' (in the construction of new knowledge)

ATTITUDINAL QUALITIES AND SELF-AWARENESS

So, in the reflective process, we learn from our experiences and also learn about ourselves. To develop as individuals, we need to get to know ourselves.

Attitudinal qualities help with our ability to reflect and gain deeper levels of self-awareness, and how this self-awareness supports and enhances reflection.

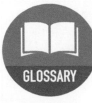

GLOSSARY

Attitude
A settled way of thinking or feeling about something: i.e. a frame of mind.

Awareness
Knowledge or perception of a situation or fact.

Attitude encompasses components that are

- Cognitive (thoughts)
- Affective (emotions)
- Motivational (enthusiasm)
- Behavioural (action)

STUDENT TIP

To reflect properly, you will need to be brave and honest with yourself.

Later on, in Chapter 8, we will see how brave Amber is when confronting her colleagues by calling out bad practice. Amber chooses to take not the easy option (and say nothing) but the professional pathway instead.

Self-awareness is the thoughtful consideration of oneself: i.e. making a conscious effort to understand and know your own

- Identity
- Beliefs
- Thoughts
- Traits
- Motivations
- Feelings
- Behaviours

We need to know how these can impact us and those around us.

It has been suggested that self-awareness is the foundation skill upon which reflection and reflective practice are built. In short, to be able to reflect, you need to know yourself. This will enable you to see yourself in a particular situation and honestly observe how you have affected the situation and how the situation has affected you. This will help you to analyse your feelings. Self-awareness is central to the ability to be:

- **Self-critical** – Critical of oneself or one's actions
- **Self-directing** – Acting freely and independently
- **Self-motivated** – Without needing pressure from others due to interest or enthusiasm

> **Tutor:** 'In one word, how did you feel after this situation?'
> **Student:** 'Fine'.
> **Tutor:** 'Now, in two words'.
> **Student:** 'Not fine'.

So, we require a level of self-awareness to be able to reflect, but do you understand how to achieve self-awareness? Two psychologists (Luft and Ingham 1955) devised a model for us to gain a better understanding; it illustrates the concept of self-awareness. This consisted of four quadrants (see Figure 1.2).

OPEN	BLIND
Known to self and to others	Not known to self but known to others
HIDDEN	**UNKNOWN**
Known to self but not to others	Not known to self or others

KEY:

The open quadrant signifies what you know about yourself and is also known to those around you.

The Blind quadrant signifies what other people know about you that perhaps you do not know about yourself

The Hidden quadrant signifies that there are things you know better about yourself that others do not

The Unknown quadrant signifies things that neither yourself or other people know about you.

Figure 1.2 Johari window.

Activity 1.1

Let's see how self-aware you are. Complete the Johari window for yourself.

LEARNING AND REFLECTION

During our training in healthcare, we may have been bombarded with reams of facts and numbers during certain lectures or training sessions. To transform what we learnt, we need to be able to make **connections** to our nursing practice. This can be achieved by reflecting on the learning contents. This will then enable us to utilise this knowledge in our nursing case studies and assignments – in short, **reflecting on what we have learned.**

Acquiring knowledge does not have to take place only through formal learning events (i.e. in the classroom), as learning is a life-wide, life-deep, life-long process. Table 1.2 shows these learning process and gives examples of each.

Another classic example of life-wide learning that all healthcare personnel adhere to, possibly without ever being taught that they are the core value and expectations of all nursing, is the 6 C's (as drawn up by NHS England):

- Care
- Compassion
- Competence
- Communication
- Courage
- Commitment

Table 1.2 Life-wide, life-deep, and life-long learning.

Life-wide learning	This teaching strategy and approach to learning and personal development involves real contexts and authentic settings. The goal is to address different kinds of learning not covered in a traditional classroom.	Example: A paediatric student nurse having difficulty getting a small child to take their medicine and asking a more experienced nurse how they manage these situations. The more experienced nurse shares her knowledge to get the child to comply.
Life-deep learning	This learning strategy refers to the social, cultural, moral, spiritual, communicational, and ethical values that lead people to act, learn, believe, and think in a particular way.	Example: A student nurse informing their tutor that they 'hate maths' whilst attending a calculations session. This is due to the student's past negative experience of learning maths whilst at school.
Life-long learning	Knowledge can be acquired and skill sets developed anywhere – learning is unavoidable and happens all the time. It is also about creating and maintaining a positive attitude to learning for both personal and professional development.	A 42-year-old hospital domestic going to evening class to obtain higher level GCSEs in order to go to university to undertake her nursing degree.

USING REFLECTION IN ASSIGNMENTS/CASE STUDIES

During your training, you will be asked to produce written assignments containing reflective practice experiences, and a more in-depth use of the reflective process will be expected. We will look at reflective assignments in Chapter 8.

Learning Journals

As a student and as part of a healthcare-related course, you will probably be expected to maintain a log/diary/journal; these are private and confidential records and usually record situations that may have actually happened to you or that you may have observed. From these written accounts, you will have evidence that you may wish to convert into a piece of critical reflection for an essay or to add to your professional portfolio. As with other reflective accounts, you should not include any confidential information in your journal, such as patient or colleague names, etc.

Learning journals usually include

- A summary of the event
- Facts relating to the incident
- Immediate learning points
- Thoughts/feelings at the time

If permitted by the learning facility, learning journals may be recorded using video diaries or audio recordings and so are not always in a written format. Following is an example of a student nurse's journal entry:

During today's shift, I was speaking to my mentor, who told me about something she had read on the wibbly wobberly web about the 15 essential skills required to pursue a career in nursing, which are said to be:

1. *Communication*
2. *Decision making*
3. *Attention to detail*
4. *Confidence*
5. *Adaptability*
6. *Physical and mental stamina*
7. *Organisation*
8. *Teamwork*
9. *Diplomacy*
10. *Leadership*
11. *Discretion*

12   *Work ethic*
13   *Interpersonal skills*
14   *Conflict resolution*
15   *Multitasking*

This got me thinking about which, if any, of these skills I have. I think I have the majority of them, but I do need to improve/work on others. I have been told that my communication and interpersonal skills are good, which I think is true. Personally, I think I am getting better at my decision-making and multitasking skills, although no mentor has ever pulled me up on these. I do need to work on my confidence skills, as I lack this and can be too hard on myself at times. I don't know about my conflict resolution skills, as I have not yet been in any conflicting situations.

This was a good exercise, as I think it really made me think about the skills I have, need to work on, and need to develop. I will keep this information and try to incorporate it in one of my course reflective assignments.

Just to note, some of the staff on this clinical placement need to work on quite a few of these essential skills!

TEST YOUR KNOWLEDGE

1   What are the 10 essential ingredients for successful reflection? Don't say 'eggs, flour', etc. – you know what I mean!
2   What are the two main types of reflection?
3   What is reflective practice?
4   The reflective process should contain six essential elements. What are they?
5   Name four benefits of reflection in nursing.
6   What are the six C's of nursing?
7   What do learning journals usually include?
8   Why do we **need** to reflect in nursing?

KEY POINTS

- Definition of reflection
- Types of reflection
- Reflective account example
- Assignment/case studies
- Reflective terminology
- The reflective process
- Why do we use reflection in nursing?
- Attitudinal qualities and self-awareness
- Learning and reflection
- Reflective assignments/case studies
- Reflective journals

USEFUL WEB RESOURCES

The 6 C's of nursing: https://nursingnotes.co.uk/resources/ the-6cs-of-nursing

NMC: www.nmc.org.uk

'Reflective practice in nursing': https://onlinelibrary.wiley. com/doi/10.1111/2047-3095.12350

Essential skills required in nursing: https://www.careeraddict. com/nurse-skills#

Agenda for Change: https://www.rcn.org.uk/get-help/ rcn-advice/agenda-for-change

Knowledge and Skills Framework: https://www.msg.scot.nhs. uk/pay/agenda-for-change/knowledge-skills-framework-ksf

NHS England: https://www.england.nhs.uk/

REFERENCES

Clarke, N.M. (2014). A person-centred enquiry into the teaching and learning experiences of reflection and reflective practice – part one. *Nurse Education Today* 34 (9): 1219–1224.

Gibbs, G. (1988). *Learning by Doing: A Guide to Teaching and Learning Methods*. Oxford: Further Education Unit, Oxford Polytechnic.

Luft, J. and Ingham, H. (1955). *The Johari Window: A Graphic Model for Interpersonal Relations*. Los Angeles, CA: University of California Western Training Lab.

Chapter 2
· · · · · · · · · · · · · · · · · · · ·
HUMAN FACTORS

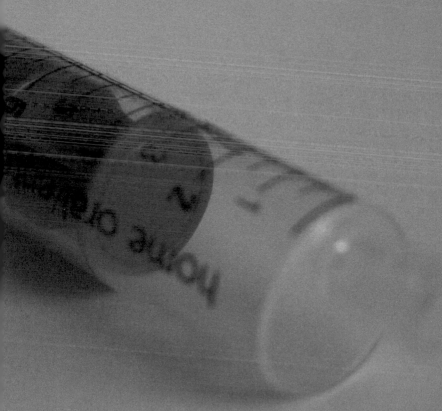

I have spoken to many nurses who informed me that they use the reflective process only when they have made a mistake and are asked by their managers to complete the process, perhaps as part of their competency proceedings action plan. These reflective accounts are usually discussed during these proceedings and/or their workplace annual appraisals.

As a confirmer for NMC revalidation, I have also had many reflective discussions with individuals using the reflection tool (Reflections Accounts form) when something went wrong in their practice. Reflection should **not** just be about the mistakes we make and the learning we acquire from analysing them, but also about the things we have done well, exploring why this was the case, and even how to make things even better.

As humans, we are not perfect (even though we may tell our partners/family/friends that we are); as such, we make mistakes and may need to improve our nursing practice. As the song goes, 'I'm only human after all, don't put the blame on me' ('Human' by Rag 'n' Bone Man). Sounds like someone is not taking responsibility!

Because we are not robots but human beings, we are fallible, and our performance at work is affected by personal life experiences, external pressures, and lack of robust support structures.

Let's be honest: healthcare can be a very stressful environment, and our working day can be quite difficult. This can lead to mistakes being made. This is where Human Factors comes in.

DID YOU KNOW?

The science of Human Factors is often referred to as 'ergonomics'.

WHAT MAKES YOUR WORKING DAY DIFFICULT?

Activity 2.1

Take a moment to think about the question 'What makes your working day difficult?'

This is a question I would often ask new employees to the trust where I worked at the time, during their induction session. These are some of the answers they gave me (do you recognise any?):

Personality clash	Poor team dynamics
Challenges	No breaks
Poor culture	Disorganisation
Poor leadership	Not sharing ideas or thoughts
Not all singing from the same song sheet	No thanks
No support/too heavy workload	Hierarchy factors at play
Low morale	Conflict
Not confident	Others taking credit for the work you do
Lazy colleagues	Demotivation
No staff	Poor attitude

By acknowledging that humans have limitations ('to err is human'), Human Factors can assess where mistakes may be made and seek to close these gaps, thus reducing error and its consequences.

DID YOU KNOW?

It has been estimated that there are approximately 850 000 adverse events per year in NHS England, costing the NHS £2 billion. It has been reported that half of these events have been thought to be preventable.

WHAT IS HUMAN FACTORS?

Human Factors really 'took off' in the aviation industry in the 1990s before being applied to healthcare!

Human Factors examines the relationship between human beings and the systems with which we interact. The focus is on improving efficiency, job satisfaction, and patient safety. The overall aim is to minimise errors. A failure to apply Human Factors principles is a key aspect of most adverse events in healthcare.

I have heard it said that healthcare workers who do not understand the basics of Human Factors are like infection control professionals not knowing about microbiology.

Here is a definition of Human Factors from Health and Safety Executive:

Human Factors refer to environmental, organisational and job factors, and human and individual characteristics, which influence behaviour at work in a way which can affect health and safety. (http://www.hse.gov.uk/humanfactors/index.htm)

HUMAN FACTORS APPLICATIONS IN HEALTHCARE

You may not have realised how deeply Human Factors has been integrated into healthcare. Table 2.1 shows some of these applications.

Table 2.1 Human Factors applications in healthcare.

To support teamwork Training in 'needs analysis' Crew resource management and Human Factors training Non-technical skills competency Assessments Checklists	In simulation Performance observation Questionnaires Physiological measures Mental workload assessment Non-technical skills assessment (situation awareness, communication, and teamwork)
In healthcare facility design Anthropometry Environmental assessment Task analysis and system modelling Prospective risk assessment Safety cases Mock-ups and prototyping Hazard identification Human reliability analysis HF-based procedure design	In technology and device design Allocation of function analysis Usability assessment Interface design and analysis Anthropometrics Mental workload assessment Task analysis and system modelling Safety cases Mock-ups, prototyping, and walk-throughs Simulation

(*Continued*)

Table 2.1 (*Continued*)

In re-organising healthcare services Task analysis and system modelling Prospective risk assessment Hazard identification Human reliability assessment Environmental assessment Workload assessment Safety cases Shift design	To support Boards to lead Safety culture and climate tools Strategic risk assessment Strategy for patient safety Error taxonomies Organisational accidents models & concepts (e.g. organisational drift) Staffing assessment Task analysis and system modelling
In allocating staffing and resources Aptitude testing Psychometric testing Non-technical skills assessment Shift design Fatigue assessment Workload assessment	In investigation and learning Interviewing techniques Investigation approaches and methods Error taxonomies Organisational accident models Safety performance measures Performance variability analysis Incident modelling
In selection and recruitment Aptitude testing Psychometric testing Non-technical skills assessment	In developing safe protocols and procedures Task analysis and system modelling Prospective risk assessment Human reliability analysis HF-based procedure design

Source: Adapted from Clinical Human Factors Group (www.cfhg.org).

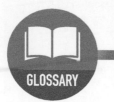

GLOSSARY

Anthropometry

The scientific study of the measurements and proportions of the human body.

WHY DO MISTAKES OCCUR IN HEALTHCARE?

Have you heard of the Swiss Cheese Effect? Imagine a stack of slices of Swiss cheese (the kind with the holes in it). All the holes are opportunities for a mistake to get through, but we have other slices to block the mistakes from getting to the

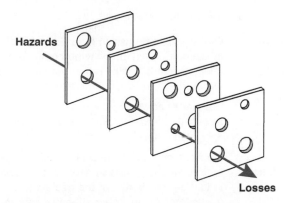

Figure 2.1 Mistake now able to get through to a patient as the holes align.

end because the holes are in different places on the slices. Each layer is a potential defence against a potential error getting to the patient. For an error to impact a patient, all the holes need to align (see Figure 2.1) – that means all our safety measures have been breached, resulting in an error.

The more defences we put up, the better, in regard to patient safety. Also, the fewer holes and the smaller these holes are, the better we are likely to catch and stop the errors that may occur. We also need to reduce the hazards, such as inadequately trained staff, staff shortages, etc. Relating this to practice, we have theatre checklists, risk assessments, etc.

Adverse Events in Healthcare

Table 2.2 shows just six of the high-profile serious incidents you may have heard about and how Human Factors contributed to the fatalities. Each and every one of these deaths represents a human tragedy – they are not just numbers but loved individuals. Each of these tragedies involved Human Factors: i.e. a catalogue of errors resulted in these patient deaths. Human Factors is about learning from our mistakes so they do not happen again. However, in the Wayne Jowett case, there had previously been 13 other **similar** mistakes (10 of them fatal) – so, are we learning?

Table 2.2 High-profile adverse events in healthcare.

Wayne Jowett – Queens Medical Centre, Nottingham (2001)	Wayne was in remission from acute lymphoblastic leukaemia. Vincristine chemotherapy drug was wrongly injected into his spine rather than intravenously. Wayne died almost one month later.
Graham Reeves – Prince Philip Hospital, Llanelli, Wales (2000)	Graham's healthy kidney was removed rather than his diseased kidney. He died five weeks after the operation.
Elaine Bromiley – xxx NHS Hospital/clinic (2005)	Elaine, a mother of two small children, underwent routine elective sinus surgery. After anaesthetic induction, intubation of the trachea was unsuccessful – repeated attempts were made but cost valuable time during which Elaine's oxygen saturations decreased to less than 40%. Difficult airway society guidelines were not followed. Elaine suffered marked brain damage and never regained consciousness.
Mid Staffordshire NHS Trust (2005–2008)	Poor care was documented, and high mortality rates were not acted upon.
Bristol heart scandal – Bristol Royal Infirmary (1990s)	Babies died at high rates after undergoing cardiac surgery. These excess mortality rates were recognised but not acted upon.
Royal Shrewsbury Hospital and Telford's Princess Royal Hospital Maternity scandal (2000–2019)	In this largest NHS maternity scandal, catastrophic failings contributed to the deaths of hundreds of babies over 20 years.

When mistakes are made in healthcare, a root cause analysis (RCA) investigation occurs, which usually leads to safety aspects being put in place, such as theatre safety checks etc., to be shared throughout the NHS.

STUDENT TIP

Mistakes are opportunities to learn and improve, so they should not just be viewed as negative.

Drug Errors

By far the most nurse reflective reports I have viewed have concerned drug errors. Let's look at some statistics: from 1 April 2015 to 31 March 2020, NHS Resolution received 1212 claims relating to errors in the medication process. Remember, this is only those making a claim, not the actual number of drug errors – i.e. only the tip of the iceberg.

DID YOU KNOW?

NHS Resolution is the operating name of the NHS Litigation Authority.

Of these claims, 487 were settled with damages paid, costing the NHS £35 million (excluding legal costs).

Activity 2.2

ACTIVITY

What do you think are the five most common medications to be implicated in incidents, according to NHS Resolution data?

If we look at NHS Resolution data, we can see that out of 146 claims reviewed that were related to drug administration errors, 'wrong route' accounted for 15% of these claims. Figure 2.2 shows a breakdown of these figures.

146 Claims Reviewed

Wrong patient	13	8%
Wrong drug	31	18%
Poor technical skills	14	8%*
Wrong dose	45	27%
Wrong route	25	15%
Delay/Omission	23	14%
Contraindicated	17	10%

* Poor technical skill, such as injection/infusion technique

Figure 2.2 Drug administration errors (1/4/2015 – 31/3/2020). From a patient safety perspective, it is important then that we learn from our drug errors to avoid them happening again.

Reflection as a Tool for Learning

Following on from the drug administration errors and the learning we can take from them, we will now look at a reflection example. (We will look at some models of reflection in Chapter 3; for your own reflection accounts, you can use whichever model you wish. Choose what works for you. We will look at the mandatory Reflective Accounts forms used in revalidation in Chapter 4.) Note that the following is an adaptation of a real-life reflective account by a registered nurse using the Gibbs Reflective Model (see Figure 2.3), which we will look at in Chapter 3.

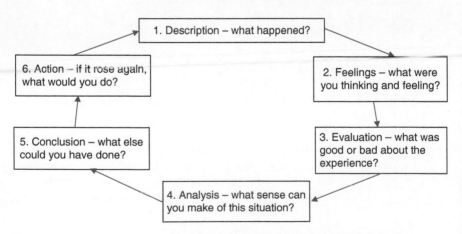

Figure 2.3 An example of a reflective account using the Gibbs Reflective Model.

1 *Drug error = Patient prescribed 600 mg co-amoxiclav IV (amoxicillin 500 mg and clavulanic acid 100 mg). Reconstituted with 10 ml water – for-injection (WFI) to be given as a bolus (preferred method) over 3–4 minutes. I did not take into account the displacement factor (0.5 mL/600 mg) whereby only 9.5 ml WFI should have been added to give the correct concentration of 600 mg/10 ml (and not 600 mg/10.5 ml). This was picked up by the second checker and corrected before administering to the patient and classed as a 'near miss'.*

2 *Felt terrible that I could have made a drug error and felt foolish.*

3 *Immediately recognised my mistake when the second checker (registered nurse) pointed out my mistake.*

4 *The clinical area was very busy with ++ staff off sick and recognised that I was taking on more work (to cover for colleagues) than I was capable of doing. Up until this time, I had worked 10 hours with no breaks.*

5 *Need to learn to delegate workload to others and not to take on more than I can manage for safe practice. Need to take allocated breaks.*

6 *Action plan has been developed: To see Practice Development Trainer to work through displacement calculations. To resit IV calculations test. Supervised drug rounds. Complete Incident form. Inform Manager and Matron. Write reflective account of incident.*

This reflective piece has some personal elements, but it reads more like a report. Points 4 and 5 could have been expanded.

TEST YOUR KNOWLEDGE

1 What is NHS Resolution?
2 What is another name for Human Factors?
3 What is the estimated number of adverse events per year in NHS England?
4 How many of these adverse events are estimated to have been preventable?
5 What is the overall aim of Human Factors?
6 What is said to be the focus of Human Factors?
7 What are the 10 main applications where Human Factors have been incorporated in healthcare?
8 What are the number of claims reviewed by NHS Resolution for drug administration errors from 1/4/2015 to 31/3/2020?

KEY POINTS

- Ergonomics/Human Factors
- What is Human Factors?
- Human Factors applications in healthcare
- Why do mistakes occur in healthcare?
- Adverse events in healthcare
- NHS Resolution
- Drug errors
- Reflection as a tool for learning

USEFUL WEB RESOURCES

Patient Safety First: Https://www.england.nhs.uk/patient-safety

Institute for Ergonomics and Human Factors: https://ergonomics.org.uk

Mid Staffordshire NHS Trust failings: http://www.gov.uk/government/publications/report-of-the-mid-staffordshire-nhs-foundation-trust-public-inquiry

Royal Shrewsbury maternity scandal: www.bbc.co.uk/news/uk-england-shropshire-60973099

Bristol heart scandal: http://news.bbc.co.uk/2/hi/health/1218149.stm

Wayne Jowett (wrong route of drug): http://news.bbc.co.uk/2/hi/health/1284244.stm

Graham Reeves (fatal kidney error): http://news.bbc.co.uk/2/hi/uk_news/wales/2041235.stm

Elaine Bromiley (just a routine operation): http://www.futurelearn.com/info/courses/airway-matters/0/steps/68647

Health and Safety Executive, Human Factors: https://www.hse.gov.uk/humanfactors/index.htm

Clinical Human factors Group: https://chfg.org

NHS Resolution, medication errors: https://resolution.nhs.uk/2022/03/31/learning-from-medication-errors

Chapter 3
· · · · · · · · · · · · · · · · · ·
MODELS
OF REFLECTION

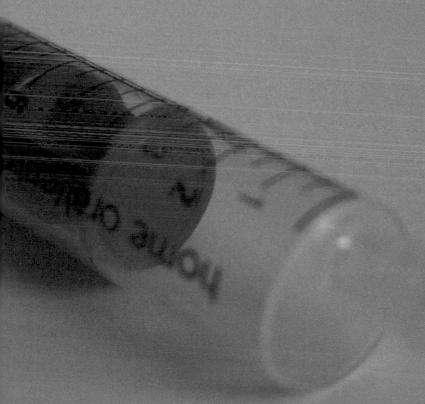

Reflective Practice for Nurses, First Edition. Claire Boyd.
© 2023 John Wiley & Sons Ltd. Published 2023 by John Wiley & Sons Ltd.

LEARNING OUTCOMES

By the end of this chapter, you should have a working knowledge of 14 models of reflection and start to understand how these models can be related to practice. You will also understand that choosing the model you wish to work with is a personal choice.

WHICH REFLECTIVE MODEL SHOULD I USE?

When it comes to reflective frameworks – there is no right model, just what works for you, because reflection is a very personal process and we all work towards it differently.

Different individuals will be drawn to different models, depending on their own preferences. You may also wish to change models as you become more of a reflective practitioner or even combine or adapt frameworks depending on the circumstances of the experience.

However, you will need to check your guidance, because as a student, you may be asked to use a particular framework for an assignment.

One key element is that all models are based on four key concepts:

- Reflection leads to learning.
- Reflection is active and dynamic.
- Reflection is progressive.
- Reflection involves viewing experiences differently.

Also, all models should enable us to think about six key elements in order for our reflection to be robust:

- Critical incident
- Description
- Analysis

- Interpretation
- Perspective
- Action

So, as we can see, models have similar traits. These frameworks can offer us structure for thinking and analysing a problem, situation, or experience, helping us to draw out learning points from this experience using a systematic approach.

We will now look at 14 models of reflection:

GIBBS REFLECTIVE CYCLE (1988)

We already had a sneaky peek at this model in action in Chapter 2. This is one of the well-known models used in nursing: it was adapted from something called the 'experimental learning cycle' and was developed to acknowledge the importance of emotions and feelings in learning.

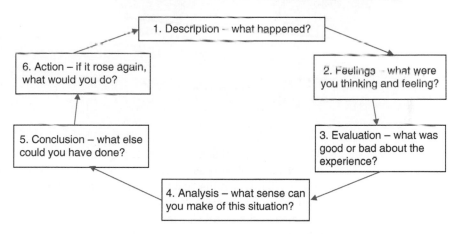

1. Description – what happened?

6. Action – if it rose again, what would you do?

2. Feelings – what were you thinking and feeling?

5. Conclusion – what else could you have done?

3. Evaluation – what was good or bad about the experience?

4. Analysis – what sense can you make of this situation?

JOHNS MODEL OF REFLECTION (1995)

This model was specifically developed for the nursing profession and is based on five cue questions that enable the reflector to break down the experience and reflect on the process and outcomes:

The Johns Model of Reflection suggests that it is important to

- Look inwards (to consider your own thoughts and feelings).
- Look outwards (to consider the experience and whether your actions were ethical and whether any external factors influenced you).

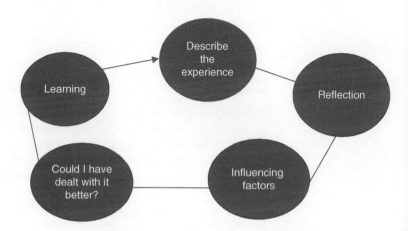

SCHÖN MODEL OF REFLECTION – BEFORE, DURING, AND AFTER ACTION (1983)

It was Schön who first proposed that professionals could use reflective thinking as a tool to improve their practice. Schön believed that the 'textbook based learning' being used to teach professionals, such as nurses, was not providing all the knowledge they required to practice effectively.

Schön's model asks these questions:

- When should we reflect on an action or activity?
- How does reflection change perspectives before, during, and after an experience?

Before an experience	During an experience	After an experience
What might be the challenges?	What's happening now, as you make rapid decisions?	What are your insights immediately after, when feelings are still fresh, and/or later, when you have more emotional distance from the event?

THE REFLECT MODEL (2015)

This model was developed by Barksby et al. in 2015 and is a modification of the Gibbs Reflective Cycle. It was developed to create a simple-to-use, easy-to-remember model using this mnemonic:

Recall the events	Stage 1: Give a brief overview of the situation on which you are reflecting. This should consist of the facts – a description of what happened.
Examine your responses	Stage 2: Discuss your thoughts and actions at the time of the incident on which you are reflecting.
Acknowledge Feelings	Stage 3: Highlight any feelings you experienced at the time of the situation on which you are reflecting.
Learn from the experience	Stage 4: Highlight what you have learnt from the situation.
Explore options	Stage 5: Discuss options for the future if you were to encounter a similar situation.
Create a plan of action	Stage 6: Create a plan for the future – this can be for further theoretical learning or action.
Set a Timescale	Stage 7: Set a time by which the plan outlined in stage 6 will be completed.

ATKINS AND MURPHY'S REFLECTIVE CYCLE (1994)

This model tends to be used by professionals who want to learn continually (shouldn't we all!).

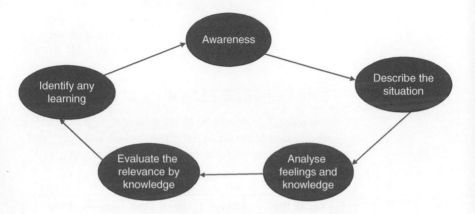

BOUD, KEOGH, AND WALKER'S MODEL OF REFLECTION (1985)

This model focuses on reflective self-analysis where the work experience must be thought about, reflected upon, and evaluated in order for personal improvement and learning to occur.

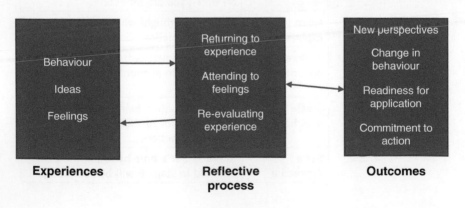

KOLB'S EXPERIENTIAL LEARNING CYCLE (1984)

Kolb suggested that effective learning is seen when a person progresses through a cycle of four stages. The learner must 'touch base' with all four stages:

Stage 1: **Concrete experience** – Learning by experience, i.e. having the experience

Stage 2: **Reflective observation** – Learning by reflection, i.e. reflecting on the experience

Stage 3: **Abstract conceptualization** – Learning by thinking, i.e. learning from the experience

Stage 4: **Active experimentation** – Learning by applying/doing, i.e. trying out what you have learned

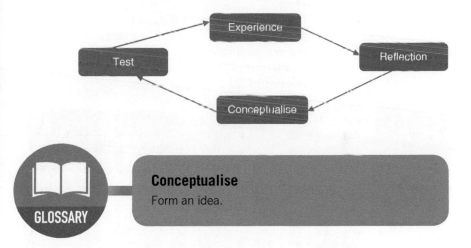

GLOSSARY

Conceptualise
Form an idea.

MEZIROW'S 10 STAGES OF REFLECTIVE PRACTICE (1983)

Mezirow's model provides a framework that helps users understand the relevance of and develop strategies for ideas, such as self-directed, experimental, practical, and applied learning, allowing users of this model to become more self-critical and more independent learners. It enables the learner to critically examine prior interpretations and assumptions to form new meaning. It is referred to as 'transformative learning', with the underpinning belief that the way we see the world affects the world. The 10 stages are as follows:

1 A **disorientating dilemma**
2 **Self-examination** with feelings of fear, anger, guilt, or shame
3 A **critical assessment** of assumptions
4 **Recognition** that one's discontent and the process of transformation are shared
5 **Exploration** of options for new roles, relationships, and actions
6 **Planning a course of action**
7 **Acquiring knowledge and skills** for implementing one's plans
8 Provisional **trying of new roles**
9 **Building competence and self-confidence** in new roles and relationships
10 A **reintegration** into one's life based on conditions dictated by one's new perspective

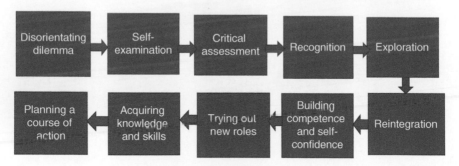

ROLF, FRESHWATER, AND JASPER'S MODEL OF REFLECTIVE PRACTICE (2001)

This model is based on three cue questions suggested by Borton in the 1970s and has been further adapted by Driscoll (2007).

This model has progressed to look at an experience, examine and consider why the observed outcome occurred, and assess personal reactions to identify how these may be improved, similar to Schön's 1991 concept of 'Reflection in Action'. Rolf et al. have referred to this as 'reflexive practice' because these questions mean we take action, which allows us to change the experience rather than just learn from it.

What?	Outline the situation (descriptive)
So what?	Discuss what you have learnt (theory and knowledge building).
Now what?	Identify the implications (action orientated).

PAAR MODEL OF REFLECTION (2008)

This model of reflection was introduced by Ghaye et al. in 2008. The abbreviations stand for 'participatory and appreciative reflection (PAAR). This model reviews what has gone well in your practice, rather than what went wrong, and therefore relates to the positive aspects of your clinical work.

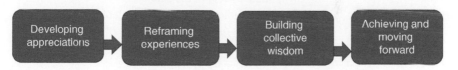

ERA CYCLE OF REFLECTION (2013)

This model was developed by Jasper in 2013 and is one of the simpler models of reflection. It consists of three steps:

1 **Experience** – Which can be positive or negative
2 **Reflection** – Thinking through the experience and examining our feelings after what happened
3 **Action** – What we do as a result of the experience, depending on our feelings and experiences leading up to it

Activity 3.1

ACTIVITY

What does the ERA in the ERA cycle of reflection stand for?

HOLM AND STEPHENSON MODEL OF REFLECTION – A STUDENT'S PERSPECTIVE (1994)

This model was developed in 1994 and is based on students questioning their roles, feelings, actions, expectations, and knowledge, as well as broader issues. It consists of a series of prompt questions to ask yourself whilst reflecting on a situation. Not all questions will be appropriate in all situations, and some questions may be asked more than once whilst reviewing:

- What was my role in the situation?
- Did I feel comfortable or uncomfortable? Why?
- What actions did I take?
- How did I and others act?
- Were my actions appropriate?
- How could I have improved the situation for myself, the patient, and my practice supervision?
- How can I change in future?
- Do I feel as if I have learned anything new about myself?
- Did I expect anything different to happen? What and why?
- Has it changed my way of thinking in any way?
- What knowledge from theory and research can I apply to this situation?
- What broader issues, for example, political or social, arise from the situation?
- What do I think about these broader issues?

STUDENT TIP

It seems that the 1980s were the decade for writing models of reflection! But even though these were developed some time ago, they stand the test of time. Why change it if it ain't broke? Personally, I like to use Kolb's Experiential Learning Cycle (1984).

WHAT ARE THE PROS AND CONS OF USING REFLECTIVE MODELS?

This question was asked to student nurses, and their answers are shown here.

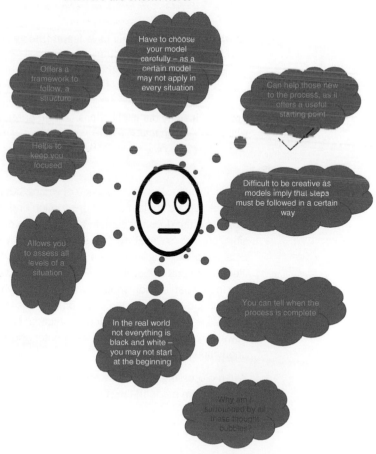

Have to choose your model carefully – as a certain model may not apply in every situation

Offers a framework to follow, a structure

Can help those new to the process, as it offers a useful starting point

Helps to keep you focused

Difficult to be creative as models imply that steps must be followed in a certain way

Allows you to assess all levels of a situation

You can tell when the process is complete

In the real world not everything is black and white – you may not start at the beginning

Why am I surrounded by all these thought bubbles?

EXAMPLE USING THE ROLF ET AL. MODEL OF REFLECTION

William, a first-year nursing student, has been asked to provide a reflective account of an incident/situation in practice as part of his course. This is his first attempt, using the Rolf et al. Model of Reflection:

What? **Outline the situation** (descriptive)

Patient on ward on bed rest due to surgery on his spine. Patient was not eating and appeared to have the beginnings of a pressure sore on his heels. Informed Mentor that patient would need to have a pressure ulcer assessment, as well as a nutritional assessment/monitoring. Also, this Mentor was in the habit of rubbing the patient's red heels 'to get the blood flowing'; I informed Mentor that this was unacceptable practice.

So what? **Discuss what you have learnt** (theory and knowledge building)

My Mentor did not like me challenging her practice and informed me that she had always done this and basically to shut up. Realised that mentor does not like me.

Now what? **Identify the implications** (action orientated)

Keep my mouth shut if I see poor practice as I want to get signed off, as a pass, at the end of this placement.

This is a very poor reflective piece of writing but a good attempt. It does contain a brief description and the student's feelings, but it does not contain an evaluation of the situation. The 'so what' section should generally be the most detailed, containing evidence and linking theory/policy/literature to practice and an action plan of the way forward. The 'now what' section should have included what this student had learnt from the situation from his research and reflections to apply this learning to practice. He had, however, remembered to keep the mentor and patient anonymous.

When discussing this course assignment with his course tutor, William made the mistake of thinking that as the model he had chosen to use was very brief, it would be quick and easy to use. He missed the point that reflection is an active process and does not just happen but requires thought and effort for learning to occur.

After talking all this through with his course tutor, William produced the following much more satisfactory reflective piece:

What? **Outline the situation** (descriptive)

Patient X was on bed rest due to his recent spinal surgery. Due to his immobility, he had been assessed as high risk on the hospital's Daily Pressure Ulcer Risk Assessment tool. I conducted his usual skin assessment (every two hours, as per protocol) and noticed redness on both heels. I conducted a 'blanch test', and as these red patches did not turn white and felt warm to the touch and slightly spongy, surmised that he had the start of pressure area problems on the heels, which I immediately informed my Mentor about. He was also not eating, and I suggested to my Mentor that this patient may need a nutritional screening and possibly a specially designed static foam mattress as opposed to the regular hospital mattress, as well as heel protectors. My Mentor looked at the heels and started rubbing them 'to get the blood flowing'; I informed my Mentor that we should never rub a suspected pressure area. My Mentor informed me that as she had been nursing for eight years, she knew better than me. She also stated that not eating for a week or two would do the patient 'no harm' as he could 'do with losing a few pounds'. My Mentor did not take kindly to my opinion and appeared quite annoyed with me for questioning her practice and was short with me for the rest of the shift, which upset me.

So what? **Discuss what you have learnt** (theory and knowledge building)

I began an evidence-based search, first on the skin massage aspect of my concern, and found that the National Institute for Health and Care Excellence (NICE) clinical care guideline (CG179), 2014 states:

1.1.10 Do not offer skin massage rubbing to adults to prevent a pressure ulcer.

1.4.10 Do not use standard-specification foam mattresses for adults with a pressure ulcer.

I also found evidence that heel protectors prevent and care for heel pressure ulcers because they completely off-load the heel and help to redistribute pressure. Pressure ulcers (decubitus) on the heels are the second most common area for bed sores to develop. Early symptoms include persistent red patches (on pale skin, purple patches on darker skin) that do not blanch (turn white) when pressed: This is known as erythema and is evidence of category 1 pressure ulcer. Other indications include when the skin feels warm and spongy – both of which this patient was experiencing. This evidence came from the European Pressure Ulcer Advisory Panel (EPUAP), 2019 (Clinical Practice Guideline (CPG), which also stated:

4.1 Conduct nutritional screening for individuals at risk of a pressure injury.

4.2 Conduct a comprehensive nutrition assessment for adults at risk of pressure injury who are screened to be at risk of malnutrition and for all adults with a pressure injury.

4.8 Offer high-calorie, high protein fortified foods and /or nutritional supplements in addition to the usual diet for adults who are at risk of developing a pressure injury and who are also malnourished or at risk of malnutrition, if nutritional requirements cannot be achieved by normal dietary intake.

The next day, I presented all my evidence to my Mentor and an action plan was drawn up for this patient, including obtaining a specialised mattress, pressure area review by specialised nurse, nutritional screening, heel protectors etc. My Mentor did not perform any more 'skin massaging' in my presence and had been sent on a Tissue Viability course.

Now what? **Identify the implications** (action oriented)

I learnt from this experience not to 'turn a blind eye' when I witnessed poor practice and to use evidence to back up my claims. Even though my Mentor did not like having her practice questioned, I had to act in the best interests of the patient and according to the NMC code: Prioritise People, Practise Effectively, Preserve Safety, Promote Professionalism and Trust.

Some of the more astute amongst you may have noticed that we have looked at only 12 models of reflection, and I had previously stated that we would be looking at 14! I wouldn't lie to you, so here are the perhaps more specific models, from the learning disabilities sector and the midwifery stated area, which you may find useful.

LEARNING DISABILITIES – MOULSTER AND GRIFFITHS MODEL

Approximately 1.5 million people in the UK have a learning disability, and people now live longer with increasingly complex health needs. This speciality of nursing lacks bespoke care models – hence the development of the Moulster and Griffiths Model (2019), which seeks to redress this shortfall and combines the reflective process with the nursing process. The model encourages nurses to reflect on their interventions at every stage:

Nursing process	Moulster and Griffiths Model	Additional elements offered by the model
Stage 1: Assessment	Stage 1: Person-centred screen Stage 2: Nursing Care Plan Stage 3: Health Equality Framework baseline	Reflection
Stage 2: Planning	Stage 4: Nursing Care Plan	Evidence base Reflection
Stage 3: Implementation	Stage 5: Nursing implementation of care plan recommendations	Reflection
Stage 4: Evaluation	Stage 6: Health Equality Framework Stage 7: Care plan evaluation	Reflection Evidence for practice

MIDWIFERY – THE HOLISTIC REFLECTIVE MODEL

The Holistic Reflective Model (Bass et al. 2017) was developed by Midwives for Midwives as an educational resource tool, with the underpinning ethos that women giving birth are not patients. The model was designed to reflect the holistic ethos of women-centred midwifery care and is similar to that of the Gibbs Reflective Cycle in that it allows for six phases of reflection through a continual learning cycle. The model embeds a conceptual continuum of reflection, critical reflection, and reflexivity, which is integral for the development of holistic reflective practice throughout the learning cycle.

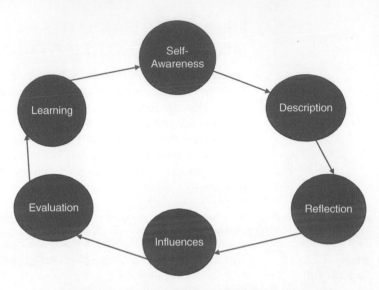

The following is an adaptation of the Holistic Reflective Model:

Self-awareness	Maintain open-mindedness to consider thoughts, responses and emotions during experience.
Description	Factual description of events, highlighting significant or important aspects.
Reflection	Thoughts and feelings explored, including underpinning values, assumptions, and beliefs to develop critical thinking skills and deeper understanding.
Influences	Draws on existing knowledge and experience (training, CPD learning, etc.) and uses a diverse range of evidence.
Evaluation	The events are objectively and critically analysed and may facilitate a change in practice.
Learning	Transformational learning, allowing the learner to synthesise and integrate the evidence reviewed during the reflection.

Source: Adapted from the Holistic Reflective Model (Bass et al. 2017).

TEST YOUR KNOWLEDGE

Think of an incident in your working life, and document it using the Rolf et al. Model of Reflection.

KEY POINTS

- Choosing a reflection model
- Gibbs Reflective Cycle (1988)
- Johns Model of reflection (1995)
- Schön Model of Reflection: Before, During and After action (1983)
- The REFLECT Model (2015)
- Atkins and Murphy's Reflective Cycle (1994)
- Bouds Model of Reflection (1985)
- Kolb's Experimental Learning Cycle (1984)
- Mezirow's 10 Stages of Reflective Practice (1983)
- Rolf et al. Model of Reflective Practice (2001)
- PARR Model of Reflection (2008)
- ERA Cycle of Reflection (2013)
- Holm et al. Model of Reflection – A Student's Perspective (1994)
- The pros and cons of using reflective models
- Example of using Rolf et al.'s Model of Reflection – good and bad
- Examples of models of reflection used in the learning disabilities sector and in midwifery

USEFUL WEB RESOURCES

Holm and Stephenson (1995) Model of Reflection – A Student's Perspective: https://www.brookes.ac.uk/students/academic-development

Rolf, Freshwater, and Jaspers (2001) Model of Reflective Practice: https://libguides.hull.ac.uk/reflectivewriting/rolfeyes

European Pressure Ulcer Advisory Panel (EPUAP):
www.epuap.org
EPUAP reference guide: https://internationalguideline.com/
static/pdfs/Quick_Reference_Guide-10Mar2019.pdf
NICE, pressure ulcers: https://www.nice.org.uk/guidance/cg179
NHS, pressure ulcers: https://www.nhs.uk/conditions/
pressure-sores
Models of reflection and reflective practice: http://London.
hee.nhs.uk/reflective-writing-models-reflection-and-
reflective-practice
**The Nursing Process and Moulster and Griffiths Model
(2019):** https://cdn.ps.emap.com/wp-content/uploads/
sites/3/2019/os/1905-A-flexible-flexible-model-to--
support-person-centred-learning-disability-nursing-pdf#

REFERENCES

Atkins, S. and Murphy, K. (1994). Reflective practice. *Nursing Standard* 8 (39).

Barksby, J., Butcher, N., and Whysall, A. (2015). A new model of reflection for clinical practice. *Nursing Times* 111 (34/35): 21–23.

Bass, J., Fenwick, J., and Sidebotham, M. (2017). Development of a model of holistic reflection to facilitate transformative learning in student midwives. *Women and Birth* 30 (3): 227–235.

Borton, T. (1970). *Reach*. Hutchinson: Touch and Teach. London.

Boud, D., Keogh, R., and Walker, D. (1985). *Reflection: Turning Experience into Learning*. London: Kogan Page.

Driscoll, J. (ed.) (2007). *Practicing Clinical Supervision. A Reflective Approach for Healthcare Professionals*. Edinburgh: Elsevier.

Ghaye, T. and Lillyman, S. (2008). *Reflection: Principles and Practice for Healthcare Professionals*. Salisbury: Quay Books.

Gibbs, G. (1988). *Learning by Doing: A Guide to Teaching and Learning Methods*. Oxford: Further Education Unit, Oxford Brookes University Press.

Jasper, M. (2013). *Beginning Reflective Practice*. Andover: Cengage Learning.

Kolb, D. (1984). *Experiential Learning: Experience of the Source of Learning and Development*. Englewood Cliffs: Prentice Hall.

Mezirow, J. (1983). *Transformative Dimensions of Adult Learning*. San Francisco: CA: Jossey-Bass.

Schön, D. (1983). *The Reflective Practitioner*. London: Temple Smith.

Chapter 4
. . . .
REFLECTION AND NMC REVALIDATION

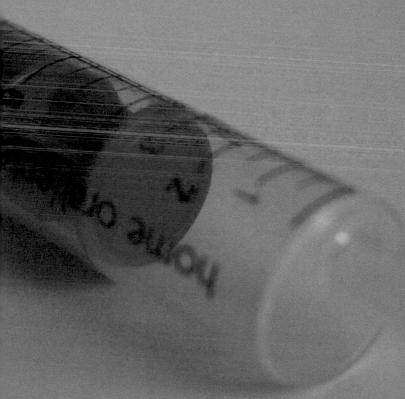

Reflective Practice for Nurses, First Edition. Claire Boyd.
© 2023 John Wiley & Sons Ltd. Published 2023 by John Wiley & Sons Ltd.

LEARNING OUTCOMES

By the end of this chapter, you should have a working knowledge of the NMC revalidation process and how to prepare a professional portfolio. You will also understand how reflection is used in areas of our working life.

Revalidation is the process all nurses and midwives in the UK and nursing associates in England need to undertake in order to maintain their registration with the Nursing and Midwifery Council (NMC). Revalidation must be completed every three years to encourage and provide evidence of continual professional development (CPD) and reflection in practice – all to promote good practice.

The NMC informs nurses, nursing associates, and midwives why we need to reflect on our practice:

> *Reflection allows you to make sense of a situation and understand how it has affected you. It allows you to identify areas of learning and development to include in your professional development objectives and support sharing and learning from other professionals. Reflective practice is a way for you to consider how you can put changes or improvements into action in your everyday practice.*

The NMC also suggests that to guide our reflective practice thinking, we should consider the following questions:

- *What key things did you take away or learn from this experience/feedback?*
- *How did you address any issues or problems that arose?*
- *What would you do differently if anything, next time around?*
- *How has it impacted on your practice?*
- *Are there any changes you can quickly apply to your practice?*

- *Are you able to support yourself or other colleagues better?*
- *What can you do to meet any gaps in your knowledge, skills and understanding?*

We are further informed that our real-life experiences should link to the four key themes of the code – which, as a healthcare professionals, we all need to abide by:

Prioritise people

1. Treat people as individuals and uphold their dignity.
2. Listen to people and respond to their preferences and concerns.
3. Make sure that people's physical, social, and psychological needs are assessed and responded to.
4. Act in the best interests of people at all times.
5. Respect people's right to privacy and confidentiality.

Practise effectively

6. Always practice in line with the best available evidence.
7. Communicate clearly.
8. Work cooperatively.
9. Share your skills, knowledge, and experience for the benefit of people receiving care and your colleagues.
10. Keep clear and accurate records relevant to your practice.
11. Be accountable for your decisions to delegate tasks and duties to other people.
12. Have in place an indemnity arrangement which provides appropriate cover for any practice you take on as a nurse or midwife in the United Kingdom.

Preserve safety

13. Recognise and work within the limits of your competence.
14. Be open and candid with all service users about all aspects of care and treatment, including when any mistakes or harm have taken place.
15. Always offer help if an emergency arises in your practice setting or anywhere else.

16 Act without delay if you believe that there is a risk to patient safety or public protection.

17 Raise concerns immediately if you believe a person is vulnerable or at risk and needs extra support and protection.

18 Advise on, prescribe, supply, dispense, or administer medicines within the limits of your training and competence, the law, our guidance, and other relevant policies, guidance, and regulations.

19 Be aware of, and reduce as far as possible, any potential for harm associated with your practice.

Promote professionalism and trust

20 Uphold the reputation of your profession at all times.

21 Uphold your position as a registered nurse or midwife or nursing associate.

22 Fulfil all registration requirements.

23 Cooperate with all investigations and audits.

24 Respond to any complaints made against you professionally.

25 Provide leadership to make sure people's well-being is protected and to improve their experiences of the health and care system.

Even if you are a student, it is good to understand the revalidation process, because you too will be using this process in the not-too-distant future! (Unless of course you are not in the healthcare profession – in which case, why are you reading this book?)

I will be honest and admit that when we first heard about the revalidation process coming into force (April 2016), there was more than a little panic in the workplace! Many of my colleagues said, 'Typical! As though we don't have enough to do!' and 'I can't even keep my professional portfolio up-to-date – when will I get time to complete all this documentation?' These same colleagues now state that they did not know what they were so worried about, as the process was far simpler than they expected and, with the NMC-provided templates, was all 'a bit of a doddle'. The reflective accounts have also helped with their practice, 'really making you think about stuff'. Could not have put it better myself!

As mentioned, all the templates are provided by the NMC and can be accessed at www.nmc.org.uk.

DID YOU KNOW?

All the NMC templates should be viewed when you are about to revalidate, as forms may have been updated.

The requirements for NMC revalidation can be seen in Table 4.1. As you can see, there is a heavy emphasis on reflection and the learning gleaned from it as part of your CPD. The reflective account should also link each event or experience to one of the four themes from the code.

Table 4.1 NMC revalidation requirements.

Documentation	Requirements
Practice hours	Minimum practice hours required for a nurse, midwife, nursing associate, nurse and specialist community public health nurse (SCPHN), midwife, and SCPHN = 450 hours. Or 900 hours if renewing two registrations, e.g. both nurse and midwife. Or 1350 hours if renewing three registration, e.g. nurse, midwife, and nursing associate
Continuing professional development	35 hours of continuing professional development (CPD) in the 3-year period since the last renewal or since the individual joined the register. Of the 35 hours, at least 20 hours must have included participatory learning.
Practice-related feedback	This can be verbal, formal, or informal and come from patients and service users, colleagues, or management. This feedback can also come from team performance reports or annual appraisals. This feedback needs to be documented.
Written reflective account	5 written reflective accounts in the 3-year period since the last renewal or since the individual joined the register.

(*Continued*)

Table 4.1 (*Continued*)

Documentation	Requirements
Reflective discussion	Reflective discussion with another NMC registrant covering the 5 written reflective accounts on the individual's CPD and/or practice-related feedback and/or an event or experience in the individual's practice and how this relates to the code.
Health and character	A declaration of health and character must be provided – fitness to practice.
Professional indemnity arrangement	Most employers provide an indemnity arrangement – individuals will need to check this. Self-employed individuals will need to arrange their own professional indemnity cover.
Confirmation	A confirmer will need to declare that the individual has met the revalidation requirement.

THE CODE

DID YOU KNOW?

The code is a set of professional standards of practice and behaviour for nurses, midwives, and nursing associates. This code used to be called 'The Code of Conduct'.

You can access the code at https://www.nmc.org.uk/code.

DID YOU KNOW?

Anonymity must be preserved on all reflective accounts.

Let me show you an example. The NMC Reflective Accounts Framework basically consists of five boxes, as you can see in this example:

Reflective account: *Witnessed poor practice*
What was the nature of the CPD activity and/or practice-related feedback and/or event or experience in your practice? *Senior House Officer (SHO) walked into c-difficile patient's room without washing hands or taking any infection control precautions e.g. apron and gloves.*
What did you learn from the CPD activity and/or feedback and/or event or experience in your practice? *That even more senior staff make mistakes and need to be reminded of Infection control policies and procedures. This SHO did not take kindly to having his practice challenged, even though this was done in a professional and courteous manner.*
How did you change or improve your practice as a result? *Aware as a nurse sometimes need to be assertive when upholding standards and values set out in the code, specially (sic) acting in the best interests of people at all times. This Doctors attitude has not deterred me from challenging poor practice in the future. After discussing the matter with this doctors Registrar, the Infection Control nurse was asked to speak to the SHO and I have now seen a marked improvement in this individuals infection control principles. I will continue to speak up when I witness poor practice, to protect patients.*
How is this relevant to the code? *Prioritise people – 4* *Practise Effectively – 6, 9* *Preserve Safety – 16, 17, 19* *Promote Professionalism and Trust – 20, 21, 22, 25*

This reflective account would have been more robust if some evidence regarding the importance of infection control protocol had been included.

DID YOU KNOW?

You can use any reflection model for your appraisal documentation and your professional portfolio. But for NMC revalidation, you must use their documentation for the **reflective accounts form,** the **reflective discussion form**, and the **confirmation form**, which are mandatory.

PROFESSIONAL PORTFOLIO

It is recommended that nurses and midwives keep a portfolio containing their professional certificates, curriculum vitae, etc. However, many healthcare professionals already keep a professional portfolio with added sections containing workplace appraisals and NMC revalidation evidence.

Here is the layout of my own professional portfolio, consisting of three sections:

Portfolio sections	What this section contains
Section 1: Personal and professional information	Name, address. NMC PIN number. Curriculum vitae (CV). Hobbies and interests. All certificates. General education and academic profile (secondary and higher education) Professional education profile (nursing degree, teaching certificate) Professional employment profile (employment history up to the present day) Continuing education and development (counselling, pain management, critical care diplomas; holistic diplomas, leadership, and management modules) Professional development planning (Master's degree) Extra information (nomination for Exceptional Healthcare Award; testimony of manager, colleagues, patients, students; author of published books for Wiley Blackwell; Freedom to Speak Guardian for the Trust, schools ambassador) Personal reflective accounts
Section 2: Work annual appraisal	Completed annual appraisal documentation
Section 3: NMC revalidation	Completed NMC revalidation documentation

This may look like a lot, but most of the input is only a line or two of writing, so the folder is actually very small. I once interviewed a qualified nurse for my team, and she brought two hefty tomes that she could barely carry – only use your professional portfolio for the essentials!

TOOLS USED IN THE REFLECTIVE PROCESS

There are many processes we use in the nursing profession that include 'reflection', such as SWOT analysis, annual workplace appraisals, 360 Degree feedback frameworks, and mind maps, to mention just a few.

SWOT Analysis

A SWOT analysis is a process that generates information that is helpful for personal and professional development, identifying your perceived strengths, weaknesses, opportunities and threats (SWOT). It is therefore useful in helping to establish which areas you may need to develop. This tool was used in healthcare as a forerunner to the reflective process, which, in all honesty, we had never heard of in the 1980s. SWOT is a useful tool and still often used in work appraisals, but it is only a data-capture exercise, as it does not include analysis. This is my SWOT analysis:

Strengths	Weaknesses
I have many years of professional experience and skills. *I can communicate effectively with team members, other managers, and patients and as a schools ambassador.* *I have been told that I have a good managerial style/am a good manager.*	*I often find it difficult to say 'no'.* *Sometimes find it hard to have difficult discussions with team members, i.e. asking them to move clinical areas in times of crisis when they do not want to go.* *Tend to work many hours over my allocated work hours: i.e. shift finishes at 21:30, still at work at 23:30.*

Opportunities	Threats
Looking into applying for my Master's degree.	As well as running a team and working full time, sometimes find it difficult balancing my work with being a schools ambassador (going to conferences and informing children about the virtues of nursing) and being a Speaking Out Guardian (for the Trust Directorate).
Work is very varied.	
Enjoy writing my nursing books and discussing contents with nursing students, nurse associates, and newly qualified nurses and midwives.	
	Have too many meetings to attend.
Enjoy teaching both 1:1 and larger groups (100+) and meeting the student nurses and spending time with them.	Team members often exhausted and stressed.
	Difficulty always finding time to mentor students.
	Staff shortages.

From my SWOT analysis, I could see that I needed to work smarter, not harder, and needed to organise some relaxation sessions for my team.

DID YOU KNOW?

SMART is an acronym and is used when goal setting:
S = Specific
M = Measurable
A = Achievable
R = Realistic
T = Timely
There are other definitions for SMART, such as 'Significant', 'Meaningful', 'Attainable', 'Reasonable', and 'Trackable'.

ANNUAL WORKPLACE APPRAISAL

Workplace appraisals are meetings between an individual and their line manager to record recent performance and achievements and to decide on future objectives. They can really make you think about your practice. Typical appraisal documentation consists of asking you to consider the following:

Your role (last 12 months)

- What are your reflections of last year, including achievements and challenges you have had
- Did you meet your objectives from last year?

Your future

- Service/Team objectives for the year ahead
- Your personal objectives for the year ahead
- Any thoughts on your longer-term career goals or plans?
- Your strengths and areas for development
- Performance development plan
- What support do you need from your appraiser/manager?

Your team

What support do you need from your manager/colleagues to achieve your objectives and goals?

Your professional responsibilities

- Are you up to date with your statutory and mandatory training?
- Have you met the core training requirements for your role?
- Are you up to date with your CPD requirements relevant for your role (e.g. NMC tri-annual review, health and safety risk assessor update training)?
- Are you on target to be eligible for your increment?

360-DEGREE FRAMEWORK (FEEDBACK)

These 'questionnaires' are designed to enable individuals to seek feedback on their leadership performance as part of the annual appraisal. The surveys usually contain the following sections about how well the individual performs, which the person giving the feedback grades from 5 = Always displays this behaviour to 1 = Never displays this behaviour. From the results, the individual can reflect on their leadership skills:

Section 1: Leadership qualities

- Communicates the vision with enthusiasm and clarity
- Challenges behaviours, symbols, and rituals that are not consistent with the vision
- Actively engages others with setting direction and service delivery
- Helps overcome obstacles and challenges in delivering the strategy
- Works collaboratively and shares information across networks
- Has an awareness of their behaviour and the impact it has on others
- Has an ability to adapt behaviour to get the best outcome in a situation
- Acts in an open, honest, and inclusive manner – respecting other people's culture, beliefs, and abilities
- Communicates clearly and effectively with others
- Listens to and takes into account the needs and feelings of others
- Ensures delivery of a safe and effective service within the allocated resources
- Balances big picture concerns with day-to-day activities
- Provides others with clear purpose and direction
- Takes action to improve performance
- Focuses self and motivates others to ensure change happens

Section 2: Improving my leadership performance

- One thing I should keep doing?
- One thing I should start doing?
- One thing I should stop doing?

MIND MAPS

Mind maps are diagrams in which information is represented visually, usually with a central idea/theme placed in the middle and the associated ideas arranged around it. Mind maps provide a structured way to capture ideas and information, helping us to see how the information fits together and supporting our thinking. An example of a simplified mind map may ask, 'What are the essential components of reflection'? Figure 4.1 shows this example.

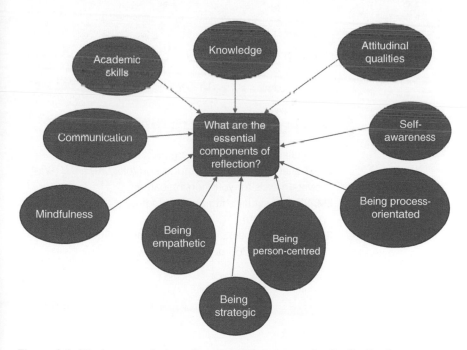

Figure 4.1 Mind map – what are the essential components of reflection?

TEST YOUR KNOWLEDGE

You may be a student nurse, a midwife, a nurse associate, or even a newly qualified nurse or overseas nurse, but you will need to revalidate with the NMC after qualification. So, it is important that you have an understanding of the revalidation process. What are the NMC revalidation requirements?

KEY POINTS

- The NMC revalidation process
- NMC code
- Example of NMC revalidation Reflective Account
- Professional portfolio
- Tools use in the reflective process
- SWOT analysis
- SMART goal setting
- Annual workplace appraisal
- 360 Degree framework feedback
- Mind maps

USEFUL WEB RESOURCES

NMC code: https://www.nmc.org.uk/standards/code
SWOT analysis: https://www.nurse.com/blog/2016/07/19/a-swot-analysis-for-your-nursing-career
SMART goal-setting: http://www.mindtools.com/pages/article/smart-goals.htm
360 Degree feedback: https://www.appraisal360.co.uk/about/what-is-360-degree-feedback

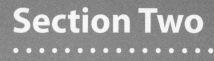

Section Two
· · · · · · · · · · · · · · · · · ·
LEARNING
THROUGH
REFLECTION

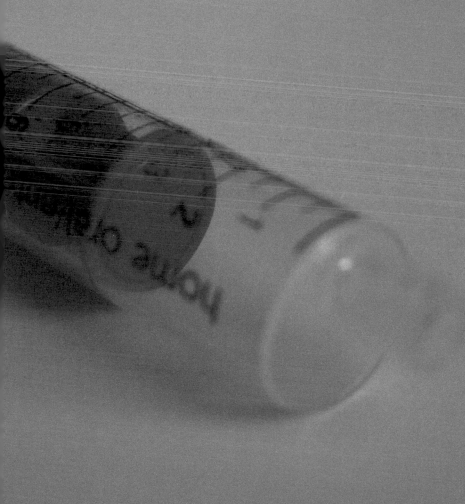

Chapter 5

WRITING REFLECTIVELY

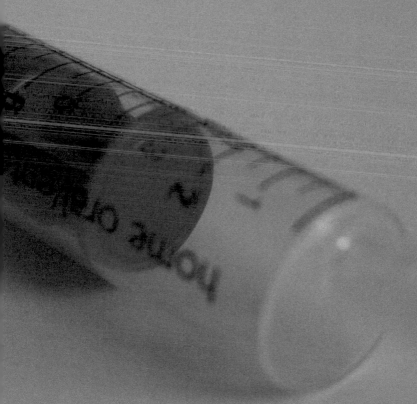

LEARNING OUTCOMES

By the end of this chapter, you should have a working knowledge of the skill of writing reflectively, distinguishing it from other forms of academic writing.

WHAT IS REFLECTIVE WRITING?

In short, reflective writing can be said to be a process of rewinding the experience and thinking about how it affected you and what you could have done differently to change the outcome and the result. You can then use this piece of reflective writing to establish what you learned from the experience and how you can apply this learning in the future. Reflection is all about you, and so is reflective writing.

One of the features of reflective writing is its specific style – often described as being 'formally informal'. Because of the personal element, reflective writing is written differently from a critical discussion, report, or literature review. It tends to use pronouns such as 'I', 'me', and 'my'. Reflective writing should carry the academic tone, being personal but not 'chatty'.

STUDENT TIP

You should always try to write in the first person when writing reflectively. This helps to focus your thoughts, feelings, and experiences rather than just writing a description of the experience.

The key to reflective writing is to be analytical rather than descriptive. It involves critically analysing an experience and recording how it has impacted you and what you plan to do with your new knowledge. Writing your experience/incident on paper helps you reflect at a deeper level due to making you think the experience through.

DID YOU KNOW?

Writing reflectively tends to move through time:
From the **past,** i.e. 'when I was', 'I felt', etc.
To the **present,** i.e. 'I find that', 'I can now see', etc.
To the **future,** i.e. 'I'd like to', 'I hope to be able to', etc.

The following table can help to distinguish what reflective writing is and what reflective writing is not:

Reflective writing generally is:	Reflective writing generally is not:
Written in the first person	Written in the third person
Analytical	Descriptive
Free-flowing	What you think you should write
Subjective	Objective
A tool to challenge assumptions	A tool to ignore assumptions
A time investment	A waste of time

WHERE ELSE IS REFLECTIVE WRITING USED?

Reflective writing can be used in many aspects of our working life and study and is therefore a skill to be achieved. You may not realise how you may have applied reflective writing in your daily life already. Here are some examples of where reflective writing can be applied:

Job applications	Many of us may be asked to show some evidence of reflection from our nursing portfolio.
Workplace appraisal	Appraisal usually contains evidence of reflection from reflecting back on the past year and showing what went well and what we need to work on due to identifying areas for improvement.
Written feedback	Many healthcare areas use the **360 Degree** feedback tool, whereby colleagues can give feedback on your performance. You may be asked to complete one of these documents.

Blogging	Blogs are a place to offer your opinion and can be a really good place to do some reflective writing. Bloggers often talk about why they like/dislike something, which can be said to be classic reflective writing.
During the research process	When we are undertaking a piece of research, we are always questioning how this project can be improved as well as different approaches to achieve the research goal in the form of reflective writing.
In academic writing	Healthcare students will be asked to include some form of reflection in an academic assignment, such as relating a topic to real-life circumstances.
In revalidation for the NMC	Nurses, midwives, and nursing associates require five reflective pieces of evidence in their portfolio when revalidating.
Learning journals	As part of a course, you may be required to maintain a log/diary/journal.

Important features of reflective writing:

- Is written in a personal manner – Using personal pronouns, such as 'I', 'me', and 'my'
- Investigates an experience in a focused manner – Using only one or two topics
- Critically analyses what has happened – Using relevant literature to link experience to theory
- Highlights implications for the future – Applying what you have learned to your future practice

STUDENT TIP

I think reflective writing is about yourself and looking back and planning forward.

As reflective writing is about writing about yourself, you may wish for a variation of constantly using the word 'I' at the start of every sentence, which may become repetitive and, dare I say it, boring! Here are some variations you may wish to consider:

Initially I . . .	It is important not to assume . . .
At first I . . .	This made me question whether . . .
In future I . . .	After reflecting on this incident, I . . .
Reflecting on this, I . . .	Looking back. . .
It became apparent to me . . .	With hindsight . . .
It was not clear to me . . .	After discussing this incident, I . . .

Reflective writing is a method of deep, self-directed learning. It helps us develop increasing self-awareness, learn from our mistakes, and challenge and change our practice, taking into account our professional responsibilities, ethical considerations, and moral obligations.

When we write reflectively, we may not abide by all the academic rules of writing; examples include reflective journals or the 'free-form' approach (which we will look at in Chapter 6). But we can still use literature to help underpin our knowledge with evidence – to reflect deeply, analytically, and critically on our experience. When we write for ourselves, it may be that no one else will see this work, but we still need to learn from these written reflections.

Reflective writing for academic purposes is quite a different creature. Writing reflectively for academic purposes can be hard, as you are expected to combine academic writing with the added element of reflection.

'I think' or 'I believe' should be used sparingly and carefully in reflective writing. However, it is useful when you are describing your own actions, decisions, or responses: 'This approach did not work, so I think I will have to try another approach next time'.

So, as you can see, there are basically two types of reflective writing:

- One for you personally – to be stored in a portfolio or journal/log and which no one else need ever read (unless you want to show it to someone you trust).
- One that is required for NMC revalidation or an assignment, case study, etc. – to be read by others (during reflective discussion or university tutor). In academic reflective writing, you will need to formalise your reflections to show that **actual learning has taken place in order to gain marks.**

BEWARE OF USING OPINIONS IN REFLECTIVE WRITING

The comments I have heard from friends (I associate with some very weird people) are sincerely held beliefs. Many think that reflection does not need to be as rigorous as other forms of writing, but you still need to supply the evidence. Otherwise, it may be meaningless – in other words, just an opinion.

When reflecting, it is absolutely fine to have an opinion, but you will need to think carefully about whether it fits in with the reflective account you are producing. Reflective writing should be about using your own personal experience as a starting point to go deeper into an issue, with your evidence then confirming or disproving the point. In short, you still need to be mindful of academic principles – to show the basis of the statements you make, with the supportive evidence. It is therefore no use being speculative without the evidence showing that aliens are indeed amongst us!

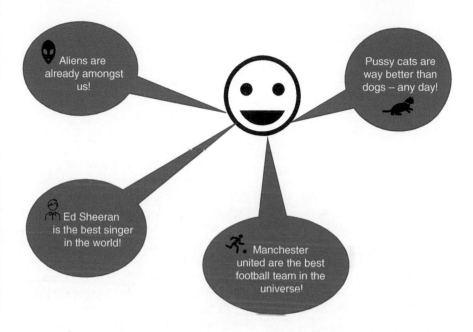

WRITING STYLE USED IN REFLECTIVE WRITING

The writing style used in reflective practice may be difficult for some to grasp, due to its differences with the more academic writing style we may be more used to. Moon (2004) sought to clarify these differences:

Undergraduate report/essay writing	Reflective writing
The subject matter is likely to be clearly identified.	The subject matter may be diffuse and ill structured.
The subject matter is not likely to be personal.	The subject matter may be personal.
The subject matter is likely to be given.	The subject matter may be determined by the writer.
The purpose of this kind of writing is set in advance, usually fairly precisely in a title/topic.	There may be purpose, but it is more in the nature of a direction, not a precise title that predicts the outcome.

Undergraduate report/essay writing	Reflective writing
Most of the ideas drawn into an essay/report will be predictable and determined by the subject matter.	Ideas will be drawn into reflective writing from anywhere that the writer believes to be relevant.
There will be a conclusion.	There may be a conclusion in that something has been learnt, or there may be recognition of further areas for reflection.
Essay/reports are more likely to be 'one off' – finished and handed in.	Reflective writing may be part of a process that takes place over a period of time.
There is likely to be a clear structure of introduction, discussion, and conclusion.	There is not necessarily a clear structure other than some description at the beginning and some identification of progress made.
The writing style is likely to be relatively objective – probably without the use of the first person.	The writing style is likely to be relatively subjective, with the involvement of the first person.
An essay or report is usually intended to be a representation of learning.	The intention underlying reflective writing is likely to be for the purpose of learning.
An essay/report is likely to be the product of a thinking process, tidily ordered.	Reflective writing usually involves the process of thinking and learning and is therefore not 'tidy' in its ordering.

Source: Adapted from Bulman and Schutz (2013) and Moon (2004).

Confidentiality is a key ethical issue in professional practice in terms of what is written and discussed (NMC 2018a).

BOLTON'S THROUGH THE LOOKING GLASS MODEL (2010)

Bolton's reflective writing model is different to the other reflective models we have looked at so far. This six-stage model is described as 'through the mirror of one's own thoughts' and is an approach to reflecting in the written format. The model enables us to discover who and what we are in practice and why we act as we do. This process may be unsettling but goes beyond ruminations and the notion that to reflect is to self-indulgently (or painfully critically) think about ourselves. You will need confidence and courage to acknowledge limitations and deficits and a degree of insight to admit these to yourself. A critical friend (stage 4) can be another student, a mentor, a tutor, or a nurse/midwife/nursing associate.

DID YOU KNOW?

Reflective/Critical conversations (stage 4) should be:

- Constructive conversations
- Helps to relate theory to practice
- Helps to identify learning
- Supportive
- Usually with a peer or whomever you feel comfortable with
- Signposts for identifying action plans (based on professional judgements)

This is a brief description of Bolton's 'through the looking glass' writing.

Stages	Explanation
Stage 1	Preparation for free writing – letting the content flow with no thought for anything else other than what we want to say on paper.
Stage 2	Free write about the experience we wish to reflect upon – do not worry about grammar, spelling, punctuation, or phrasing.
Stage 3	Read our free writing – digest the story we have written.
Stage 4	Find someone we trust to read our free writing – ask them to act as our external critical friend. This is called the 'reflective conversation'.
Stage 5	Become reflexive – writing about the same experience from a different point of view. See how our experience impacted those around us, to provide us with a different perspective.
Stage 6	After reflecting deeply – prepare our reflective writing for academic purposes (if there is a requirement to do so), going through the content and formatting, shaping and reworking the information into a piece suitable for academic purposes.

DID YOU KNOW?

Free writing: Bolton describes this as 'dumping mind clutter onto paper'. Some of this may only be scurrilous moans, but the important thing is to allow the writing to follow its own track. Write whatever is in your head, keeping it uncensored. Whatever is written will be right, as it is yours – no one else ever needs to read it, if you don't want.

Through-the-looking-glass reflection can facilitate:

Gaining perspective	Giving confidential and relatively safe access	Releasing power to take more responsibility for actions	Using narrative, which offers accurate observation, metaphor, and critique

The process of reflection writing involves considering the meaning and impact of an experience, which enables learning about yourself both personally and professionally.

Here is an example of Bolton's free writing from the Through the Looking Glass Model of reflective writing (stages 1–3):

X was due to deliver a presentation trust wide. Participants had started turning up and the room was not ready. Even though I was +++ busy on the ward, I thought that I would set up for her as an act of kindness and to help her out. I had almost completed the task and with 5 mins to go before the presentation was due to start, X stormed into the room and shouted at me as to why the room was not ready!! This was done in front of ++ participants and left me feeling humiliated and angry. I threw the handouts on the nearesr dest and left the room. Another colleague came up to me, seeing I was upset. We talked through the situation that had just occurred, and how this other colleague had been rude to me, and my colleague reminded me that it was not in X's nature to ever say 'thank you' and she was particularly bad natured at present due to her partner being in hospital due to health problems, which made sense to me. I was undecided whether to tell X that she should have been thankful that I had helped her out of a hole and that I did not deserve to be treated in that manner. I have decided not to take X's unprofessionalism to heart and to be more understanding of X's personal situation. I will however discuss this incident with X, explaining how her actions had made me feel, in order to clear the air and as a means to moving forward with our professional relationship. I do think that X needs to be more mindful of her rude behaviour.

As we can see from this piece of free writing, there are a scattering of spelling mistakes. This is the essence of free writing – just going with the flow. The writer could then continue with stages 4–6 of this model.

REFLECTIVE DISCUSSION

Reflective discussions can be used in lots of different ways, such as

- To share ideas, information, and experiences
- To debrief after an incident
- To get another person's perspective on a situation
- To think about professional development objectives

Activity 5.1

ACTIVITY

Think of an incident in your work environment, and try some free writing to de-clutter the incident from your mind. Remember, no one needs to see this writing unless you want them to.

COMMON MISTAKES IN WRITING REFLECTIVELY

Writing reflectively is a learned skill for many individuals in the world of academia. This is because we may focus too much on describing the experience. Following are some phrases that may assist you in avoiding this situation and that can be used in the main body of your reflective piece or the conclusion/plan of actions:

The most important thing was . . .	Later I realised . . .
At the time, I felt . . .	This was because . . .
This was likely due to . . .	This was like . . ..
After thinking about it . . .	I wonder what would happen if . . .
I learned that . . .	I'm still unsure about . . .
I need to know more about . . .	My next steps are . . .

Here are some more useful words and phrases that can be used in the conclusion of your reflective writing and for your plan of actions:

Conclusion			
Having	read	I now	feel
	experienced		think
	applied		realise
	discussed		wonder
	analysed		question
	learned		know
		Additionally	I have learnt that
		Furthermore	
		Most importantly	
I have (not)	significantly	developed	My skills in
	slightly	improved	My understanding of
			My knowledge of
			My ability to
This means that			
This makes me feel			
The knowledge	is	essential	To me personally because
This understanding	could be	important	To me as a student because

Conclusion			
This skill	will be	useful	To me as a nurse/ Midwife
ACTION PLAN	Did not		
This means that			
This makes me feel			
The knowledge	is	essential	To me personally because
The understanding	Could be	important	To me as a student because
The skill	Will be	useful	To me as a nurse
	Did not		
	Have not yet		
	Am not yet certain about		I now need to
	Am not yet confident about		
	Do not yet know		
	Do not yet understand		
			As a next step I will

Source: Adapted from Dalves-Yates (2021).

Activity 5.2

ACTIVITY

How not to write reflectively: Elliot works in a residential care home and wrote his reflective piece using **text talk** when using the Rolf et al. Model of Reflection. What the heck does it all mean?

What?	I did not check SU BG B4 admin. Insulin 😔
So what?	AFAIK this can be Srsly dangerous if SU's BG is very low & NSFL. FYI instead of insulin, in this 💼 they require glucose 🍔 ASAP
Now what?	Ngl, TIL I need 2 follow CH protocol. I will always check BG from now on 😊

Just to note, text talk like this should never be used in practice to complete reflective accounts.

EXAMPLE USING KOLB'S EXPERIENTIAL LEARNING CYCLE MODEL (1984)

Now we will look at putting Kolb's Experiential Learning Cycle Model into practice. Wani is a senior staff nurse who took a venepuncture sample and forwarded it to the pathology laboratory in a yellow sample bag. Amber, a health care assistant (HCA), informed Wani, in a courteous and professional manner, that the sample should have been forwarded to the lab in a red sample bag, as per protocol.

Stage 1: Concrete Experience – Learning by experience, i.e. having the experience

I had taken the requested venepuncture sample from patient X and labelled the sample tube. I then proceeded to put this sample, with the required documentation, into a yellow specimen bag and sealed this bag in order to forward to the Pathology Laboratory. My co-worker, a Health Care Assistant informed me that this was the wrong specimen bag, as the correct specimen bag was the red one.

Stage 2: Reflective Observation – Learning by reflection, i.e. reflecting on the experience

My initial feeling was that I did not like being told how to do my job by a HCA, especially since I had been performing this skill for many years, which I informed the HCA (possibly in an angry manner). I had always put venepuncture samples in whatever bag was to hand. Bags come in a variety of colours – it does not matter whichever colour sample bag the sample is placed.

Stage 3: Abstract Conceptualization – Learning by thinking, i.e. learning from the experience

I decided to check the venepuncture policy and Pathology protocol and was informed:

'Individual samples must be in sealed appropriately coloured specimen bag. Samples for separate pathology departments must not be placed in the same specimen bag, failure to separate samples appropriately at collection will cause unnecessary delay in the laboratory. Sample bags:

Blood Sciences – Red Specimen Bag (Clear Specimen bag if red specimen bag not available)

Infection Sciences – Blue Specimen Bag
Histology – Yellow Specimen Bag
Cytology – White or White/Purple Specimen Bag
Genetics – Clear Specimen Bag'

I was shocked at this information as I had been sending samples in wrong coloured specimen bags. Also, I had never seen a white/purple bag, and did not know they even existed.

I organised a visit to the Pathology Lab and found that in the Lab an Assistant gathers up the samples from the pneumatic tube (forwarded from the clinical areas in the main hospital) and separates each colour bag and forwards those samples to different parts of the Lab. Therefore, my venepuncture samples, placed in a yellow bag, go to the histology section of the lab and it could be some time before an Assistant takes the venepuncture samples from the Histology section to the Blood Sciences section, therefore delaying the patient results. I felt embarrassed by my mistake.

Stage 4: Active Experimentation – Learning by applying/ doing, i.e. trying out what you have learned

I realised that due to the hectic work pace due to covid and winter pressures, it was no excuse to not keep updated with my skills, which I now intend to exercise. I will also in the future need to be mindful and abide by the Nursing and Midwifery Council Code, specifically:

Practise Effectively:
6. Always practice in line with the best available evidence
8. Work co-operatively
8.1 Respect the skills, expertise and contributions of your colleagues, referring matters to them when appropriate

8.4 Work with colleagues to evaluate the quality of your work and that of the team

8.6 Share information to identify and reduce the risk.

What do you think about this piece of reflective writing? My concern is, where is Wani's apology to the HCA, Amber, and the recognition that she showed anger to this co-worker, who was in the right? This lack of respect could undermine any cohesive team working as Amber may be afraid to challenge any poor practice in the future. Wani paid lip service to the NMC code but did not actually practice what she wrote, specifically section 8.1.

TEST YOUR KNOWLEDGE

Think of an incident in your working life, and document it using Kolb's Experiential Learning Cycle Model of Reflection.

KEY POINTS

- Components of reflective writing
- Where reflective writing is used in everyday situations
- Important features of reflective writing
- How to compare reflective writing with report/essay writing
- Bolton (2010) Through the Looking Glass Model of reflective writing
- Reflective discussions
- Useful words and phrases to be used in reflective writing
- Example of Kolb's Experiential Learning Cycle (1984)

USEFUL WEB RESOURCES

Jenny Moon, reflection: https://www.cemp.ac.uk/people/jennymoon/reflectivelearning.php

Jenny Moon, reflective learning: https://www.cemp.ac.uk/people/jennymoon.php

NMC, standards of proficiency for registered nurses:
http:www.nmc.org.uk/standards/standards-for-nurses/
standards-of-proficiency-for-registered-nurses
NMC, standards of proficiency for registered nursing associates: https://www.nmc.org.uk/standards/
standards-for-nursing-associates/

REFERENCES

Bolton, G. (2010). *Reflective Practice: Writing and Professional Development*, 3e. London: Sage.

Bulman, C. and Schutz, S. (2013). *Reflective Practice in Nursing.* 5th Edition, Oxford, Wiley-Blackwell.

Dalves-Yates, C. (2021). *Beginner's Guide to Reflective Practice in Nursing.* London: SAGE Publications Ltd.

Kolb, D. (1984). *Experimental Learning: Experience of the Source of Learning and Development.* Englewood Cliffs: Prentice Hall.

Moon, J.A. (2004). *A Handbook of Reflective and Experiential Learning.* London: Routledge Falmer.

Chapter 6

· · · · · · · · · · · · · · · · · · ·

IMPROVING CARE THROUGH REFLECTION

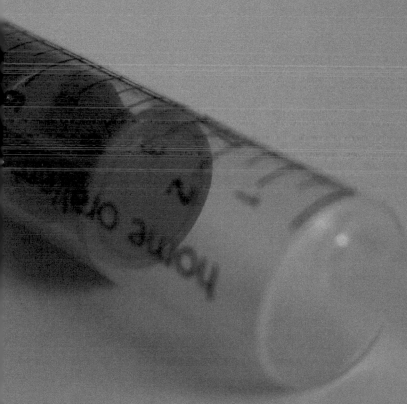

Reflective Practice for Nurses, First Edition. Claire Boyd.

LEARNING OUTCOMES

By the end of this chapter, you should have a working knowledge of how reflection is linked to improving care in clinical practice.

Many years ago, I was asked to write a nursing assignment using the Gibbs Reflective Cycle (1988), for a course I was on, and one thing I learnt from this exercise was that I did not like using this model for the incident I wished to write about! I felt some of the stages were unclear, and some repeated themselves. Today there are many models to choose from: some are over-simplified, allowing the reflector to approach the process in a superficial way, whilst others are overly complex. I can work out Einstein's Theory of Relativity $E = MC^2$ more easily than I can use some of these models! (O.K., that was a lie – just been on the internet and don't understand a word of it!)

STUDENT TIP

Always read the assignment brief, as you may not get the choice of which model to use – choosing your own reflective model to use instead of the specified one will affect your grades.

DO I HAVE TO USE A REFLECTION MODEL?

So what can you do if you have a choice for a reflective model and don't want to use any you have seen so far – i.e. if you don't feel comfortable using any of them as they do not fit with what you want to write about?

I have often been asked, 'Do I have to use a model of reflection?' The answer is, if you can't find a model you like or wish to use, you can go freestyle – as long as the reflection you are writing about contains all the elements a reflective piece should contain (see Chapter 5).

Activity 6.1

Think back to Chapter 5. What are the important features of reflective writing?

*
*
*
*

Even better, you can adapt an existing model or even combine elements of two or more reflective models that include the relevant parts, to help you produce your piece of reflection. However, you will need to be mindful that a course assignment may specify that your **reflection should use a specific model of their choosing**. Also, in the NMC revalidation process, you need to use the Reflective Account documentation.

If you do wish to go down the free style/ 'free form' route, just thinking and seeing where this takes you, and not following a structured model approach, this is fine for your own personal reflective accounts.

DID YOU KNOW?

When you produce a reflective account, you can choose to use either a structured model or a free-form approach. 'Free-form' just means an unstructured approach.

I mentioned in Chapter 1 that I tend to use my own reflection model when reflecting on my personal incidents/ experiences; it has elements of free-form and a loose structure. I always start off with a description, and the other elements appear somewhere in the contents! I also tend to look at the past, present, and future aspects in the reflective piece, as seen here:

This is what happened	PAST
How do I feel?	
Could I have done anything differently? (analysing)	PRESENT
Planning a course of action (exploration)	
What I have learnt – acquiring knowledge and skills (life-long)	FUTURE

Free-form approach

Structured model approach

Free spirits this way

HMS Tight Ship this way

Free-form is not without value for your personal learning, as you are not limiting yourself to answering a particular set of predefined questions. However, we all need to remember that personal reflections still need to uphold the definition of 'reflection', i.e. the important features of reflective writing; otherwise, this process just produces 'writing' and not 'reflection'.

STUDENT TIP

Do not get muddled up between **free Form** (writing) and **free from** (gluten-free, dairy-free, etc. foods) – just saying!

The following is an example of free-form reflective writing from a health care assistant (HCA), written as part of a course she was attending. She was asked to reflect on how her presentation to her peers had gone:

Reflection on my presentation

I decided to do my presentation on 'Feeding the newborn' as I work very closely with mothers and their babies in this hospital area. I also feel very passionate about breastfeeding and helping and supporting mothers in achieving and managing this natural process correctly.

I was very nervous at the start, and asked to deliver my presentation first, to get it over and done with, so my nerves wouldn't get any worse whilst I was waiting to deliver the presentation.

My talk began by firstly talking about myself and what I was going to be talking about. This was my introduction. I then started with the big benefits of breastfeeding that I thought were important. I then explained the health benefits for mothers and their baby. I included this as I felt that not many mothers actually realise the benefits that they can get from breastfeeding. I included a lot of pictures and colours as I find they help get the information across easier and are more interesting to look at. I then talked about the negatives of breastfeeding as I didn't want women to think breastfeeding was easy as it can be hard work and a lot of effort is needed. I then talked about the different sign posts to look for when out-and-about and places to go when out where they can breastfeed, as a lot of women aren't aware that many places welcome breastfeeding.

I then went on to talk about formula feeding and looked at the disadvantages and advantages of this. I thought I would include this as many mothers do formula feed and wanted to show both sides of the story for some balance, and that as long as their baby is happy and healthy it doesn't really matter what you feed them.

I feel that my presentation went well, although I know I did get flustered at one point of the presentation and was aware that I needed to slow down as I was talking too fast and higher than normal. I think that I should have given a little more information on formula feeding, but I support breastfeeding in my day-to-day life and felt it was very difficult to give encouraging information about formula feeding. If I did my presentation again I think I would add some information on expressing and sterilising as I then can give advice on the correct procedure for doing this. I also think that I should have asked if anyone had any questions at the end of the presentation.

As you can see from this first excellent attempt at reflective writing, this HCA built in

- Her experience
- An evidence base
- Her feelings
- Moving forward

Or:

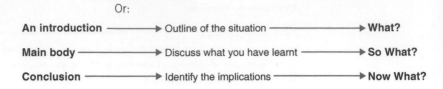

An introduction ⟶ Outline of the situation ⟶ **What?**

Main body ⟶ Discuss what you have learnt ⟶ **So What?**

Conclusion ⟶ Identify the implications ⟶ **Now What?**

In other words, she was using the Rolf et al. Model of Reflection without even knowing it!

Note that the comment *'as long as their baby is happy and healthy it doesn't really matter what you feed them'* is not strictly true, as this is an opinion without academic evidence.

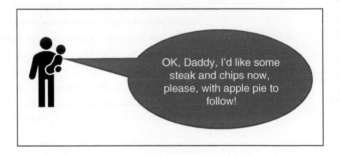

Barriers to Reflection

When I asked a cohort of student nurses to share their reflective accounts, a couple of these students informed me that they felt too embarrassed to share. I agree absolutely, as I have some written pieces I would not want to share – for my eyes only, my own personal reflective accounts. We do not need to share our own personal reflections with anyone.

This also brought about the discussion about how honest these students could be in their reflections as part of a graded assignment or as part of a demonstration of achievement of outcomes in practice settings. I was informed that this has led to these students writing what they believe their tutors and mentors **want** to read and what they think will generate higher grades, instead of writing about what actually happened.

This was also true when discussing the NMC revalidation reflective accounts with nurses – I was told that nurses often only write about what they think will look better to their manager (or NMC confirmer) – not their true accounts. Reflection should be about learning to be the best we can, and we should not forget that **reflective practice is considered an essential aspect of improving nursing care** – honesty should be paramount, but it can be easily seen why we may want to dilute this experience.

Other barriers to reflection, according to the student nurses, were

- Not seeing the relevance of reflection, and therefore a lack of motivation
- Not fully understanding how to reflect
- Tiredness after a heavy shift or day of lectures
- Lack of time to reflect
- Distractions – can't find a quiet space to reflect on the day's events
- Can't reflect on a specific incidence as it brings back bad memories
- Not able to see the relevance or link between the reflective process and learning

As students progress in their nursing career and use reflection in their practice more frequently, the benefits of reflection do become more apparent.

Another discussion involved when to use reflection: when we make mistakes? or when something good happens in practice?

REFLECTION – THE POSITIVES AND THE NEGATIVES

Recently, talking to a group of brand-new student nurses embarking on their nurse training, I asked them what 'reflection' meant to them. Although some did state that they were aware reflection was 'part of the revalidation process' and 'helps us to become better at our job', many only saw the revalidation process in the negative, with comments like these:

- Performed only when you make a mistake
- Mainly used by students as part of their nursing assignments
- Undertaken only when told to
- Performed as part of the capability process

These students were shocked to find out that reflection can be used in the positive – i.e. when things go right – to reflect on why this was the case and what to do to make the experience/situation even better. In short, **reflection in practice is about learning, and according to the NMC:**

- It ensures nurses and midwives act on their learning.
- Reflecting on practice increases self-awareness and motivation to make improvements.
- Reflection allows the code to become the focus of practice and improves the standards of care delivered to patients.

NMC REFLECTIVE ACCOUNT

The following reflection is an account by a nurse who has been qualified for over 20 years and went on a training event about dementia. This nurse came away from the training event delighted that she had learnt so much about a topic she thought she already knew a good deal about. This goes to show that reflection can be about positive events, and we are all life-long learners!

What was the nature of the CPD activity and/or practice-related feedback and/or event or experience in your practice?

I attended a training event on Dementia, and found this session very useful. Really understood the analogy of memory loss and the wobbling bookcase. Relating the tall unstable bookcase to a person helped me to understand this condition much better.

What did you learn from the CPD activity and/or feedback and/or event or experience in your practice?

Why dementia sufferers forget about events from their recent memory first and retain memories from years ago – which I found very interesting: As the unstable bookcase wobbles, books from the top shelves fall away first and the lower down books on shelves stay in place (i.e. Top shelf = now, lower shelves = childhood/past). This occurs as areas of the brain responsible for these memories become damaged. Also explains why individuals retain emotional memories – but may not know why they have these feelings and emotions – again due to different parts of the brain affected.

Learning about dementia was very interesting and has made me want to learn more about this condition.

How did you change or improve your practice as a result?

This session gave me a better understanding of the dementia process and the devastating effects of this to the individual person. This understanding enables me to be more tolerant to their condition. I will certainly apply what I have learnt today in my clinical practice. I intend to give a brief presentation to my colleagues of what I have learned today during the next team meeting – sharing my knowledge.

How is this relevant to the code?
Select one or more themes: Prioritise people – Practise effectively – Preserve safety – Promote professionalism and trust

Prioritise people – 1, 2, 3, 4,

Practise effectively – 6, 7, 8, 9

LIFE-LONG LEARNERS

As life-long learners, we can always improve our practice. Some of us may feel that we don't need to improve our reflection skills – really?! The Royal College of Nursing (RCN) have produced tips to improve our reflection for revalidation, but they can be utilised by any of us wishing to use the reflection process. See Table 6.1.

REFLECTIVE LEARNING

Reflective learning involves actively monitoring and assessing your knowledge, abilities, and performance during the learning process. This is to improve the process and its associated outcomes.

Table 6.1 RCN tips to improve your reflection.

Get in the habit of reflecting on your work.	The sooner, the better, as your memories are fresher; this will also ensure a more truthful account. Jot down a couple of bullet points, perhaps on your phone if you don't have time at the moment to write them down.
Think about when you avoid reflection.	You may find it difficult to write down your feelings or articulate your experiences. Choose a reflective model that works for you, or draw word clouds or illustrations, before adding the meat to the bones at a later time to complete the process.
Identify what you are good at.	Reflection is about making changes to enhance your practice, so you will need to identify a combination of events to reflect on – some that were positive and some that challenged you.
Structure your learning across three years.	Avoid leaving your revalidation to the last minute – keep reviewing your reflective pieces and adding your CPD evidence throughout the three years.
Make the most of learning events.	Keep learning and compiling evidence of these learning events.
Keep your portfolio up-to-date.	Find a regular time to organize your portfolio, perhaps once every two months.
Familiarise yourself with the code.	Reflective accounts need to be related to the NMC code, so when recording your reflections, make sure you are familiar with the code contents, linking your practice to the four themes.
Show what you have learned.	Use the templates provided by the NMC to record all your CPD hours, reflections, etc. Keep these in a safe place.

Source: Adapted from RCN 'Eight ways to improve your reflection'.

An example of reflective learning may be when we are asked to write an assignment and find we are struggling with it – we ask ourselves why and try to figure out what reading we may need to undertake to rectify this situation. We may think about talking to our tutor and/or peers. This is also where our reflective logs may give us inspiration.

The benefits of reflective learning are as follows:

- It can help you assess your situation – prompting you to identify gaps in your knowledge and areas you may need to improve.

- It can help you to improve your learning process – helping you identify which learning techniques work well for you and which don't.
- It can help you better understand yourself – prompting you to consider which kind of assignments/information you struggle with most.
- It can help you develop your general metacognitive skills – training you to think critically about how you learn.
- It can increase your feelings of autonomy and control – helping you feel in charge of the learning process.
- It can increase your motivation to learn – helping you feel more in control of the learning process and making this process more effective.
- It can improve your learning outcomes – helping you modify the learning process.

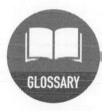

GLOSSARY

Metacognitive skills
Awareness and understanding of our own thought processes.

Autonomy
Freedom from external control or influence; independence.

Studies have shown that reflective learning can lead to personal growth and improved learning, also helping students to process the learning material and link it to material that they have encountered previously. Reflective learning has also been found to improve our critical thinking skills and the ability to organise our thoughts.

Being a reflective learner means thinking about what you're learning and how you are learning it. In your learning, you can reflect on

- Your understanding of the material – how well you understand certain concepts
- Your understanding of how to implement what you've learned – putting this learning into clinical practice

- Your learning process – how well certain learning strategies work for you
- Your abilities, preferences, and thoughts – how difficult or enjoyable you may find certain topics, e.g. nursing calculations
- Your goals – what you hope to achieve by implementing what you have learned

Reflective learning can be quick and shallow or slow and deeper:

Quick and shallow reflective learning: when studying, you may ask yourself . . .	Slow and deeper reflective learning: when studying, you may . . .
'Do I really understand this material?'	You may want to write down all the key points you learned about and go over this list to identify areas you may not have understood so well.
'Is this learning technique working well for me?'	You may decide to write down a list of all the learning techniques you are using and then rank them based on how effective they are for you.

Reflective learning can be a shared activity, something you can undertake on your own or together with others. This can take many forms, such as a group of nursing students discussing the challenges they all face while studying for a calculations test or a one-to-one meeting between a student and a tutor where the tutor asks the student guiding questions about the students learning process. Shared reflection has positives and negatives:

Shared reflection – advantages	Shared reflection — disadvantages
Exposes people to more perspectives, which can help them identify more issues with their learning than they would be able to identify in a pair or by themselves.	A shared approach can be stressful for people who are shy and don't like to speak up in larger groups.

LEARNING IN PRACTICE

Even when mistakes occur in healthcare (remember Human Factors from Chapter 2?), we still need to use these situations as learning events.

Unfortunately, in healthcare, medication errors occur frequently. Medication errors are among the most common health-threatening mistakes affecting patient care. Such mistakes are considered a global problem that increases mortality rates, length of hospital stays, and related costs.

Human Factors (see Chapter 2) may affect the incidence of nursing medication errors for these reasons:

- Hectic shift/too busy
- Too tired and unable to take breaks
- Staff shortages
- Workload too heavy
- Inadequate training of staff
- Incorrect medicinal calculations
- Lack of pharmacological knowledge

Figure 6.1 shows the back of two drug packages, which look very similar. In a busy environment, these drugs could be grabbed, mistaken for the same drug, and administered without due care and attention.

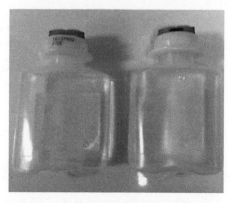

Figure 6.1 The back of two medication packages.

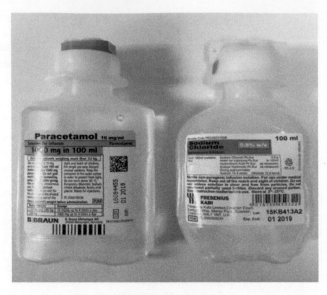

Figure 6.2 The front of the two medication packages.

On the other hand, Figure 6.2 shows the fronts of these medications. We can see that they are two completely different medications.

In short, no matter how tired or rushed we are, we need to concentrate when administering medication, as we have seen how easy it can be to make a mistake – in this case, picking up the wrong container. Drug administration requires thought and professional judgement.

If we do make a medication error, we will usually be asked to produce a written reflective account, perhaps as part of the capability process.

TEST YOUR KNOWLEDGE

Think of the last learning event you attended, and reflect on it using the NMC Reflective Account questions:

1 **What was the nature of the CPD activity and/or practice-related feedback and/or event or experience in your practice?**

2   What did you learn from the CPD activity and/or feedback and/or event or experience in your practice?
3   How did you change or improve your practice as a result?
4   How is this relevant to the Code?

KEY POINTS

- Adapting models of reflection
- Free-form reflection
- Barriers to reflection
- Reflection – the positives
- Reflection – the negatives
- NMC Reflective Account – example
- Life-long learners
- Tips to improve reflection
- Reflective learning
- Learning in practice
- Medication errors

USEFUL WEB RESOURCES

NMC: www.nmc.org.uk
RCN tips for improving reflection for revalidation: https://www.rcn.org.uk/professional-development/revalidation?

Chapter 7

- - - - - - - - - - - - - - - - - - -

CRITICAL
REFLECTION

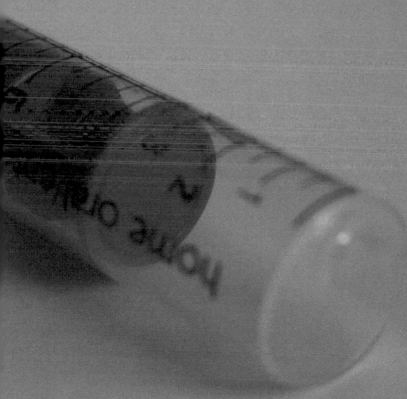

Reflective Practice for Nurses, First Edition. Claire Boyd.

LEARNING OUTCOMES

By the end of this chapter, you should have a working knowledge of critical reflection and how this differs from description and reflection. You will also have an understanding of critical incidents, critical reflection models, and critical thinking.

WHAT IS CRITICAL REFLECTION?

Critical reflection is an effective means of engaging in professional and personal development through self-assessment and self-evaluation. It is also a means of looking at the quality of practice and questioning how things are done.

By using critical reflection, nurses can develop a better understanding of the ways in which we all practice, the influences on our practice, and our responses to challenging situations and reflection on critical incidents: specifically, questioning our practice and demonstrating our ability to

- Explore, question, and analyse your experiences.
- Use your knowledge to enhance your understanding of these experiences.
- Use your knowledge to shape your future experiences.
- Learn from past experiences, assess options and make decisions in presenting scenarios, and implement changes or routines to ensure that future experiences will improve.

All reflection can be said to be 'critical' as this simply means **critical thinking**. However, there are some subtle differences. Critical thinking is central to reflection and becoming a reflective practitioner and can assist you in

- Making those difficult decisions
- Justifying practice
- Identifying how you have arrived at your decisions (based on a sound knowledge base)

The terms 'critical' and 'reflective' can be combined to produce the term 'critical reflection', meaning the reflector has thought carefully about an incident or situation. To be critical, you have stepped up this process a notch.

There are two key differences between critical and reflective writing. Reflective writing is more about:

1 **Thinking processes at work**
   You and your thinking are more visible in your writing.

2 **Going on a personal journey**
   Looking at what you have done, thought, and read; the changes you will make along the way; and what you will do next.

Chapter 14 will show these processes in action.

CRITICAL INCIDENTS

Critical reflection can be part of a capability process, whereby someone has made a mistake and their work is under review. As part of this process, they may be asked to produce a piece of reflection regarding the mistake – a critical reflective piece or critical incident analysis. It should be noted that, critical incident analysis can be applied to both positive and negative situations, as we have discussed previously.

Activity 7.1

Can critical incident analysis be applied to both positive and negative situations?
Note: You may want to re-read the last sentence before this activity!

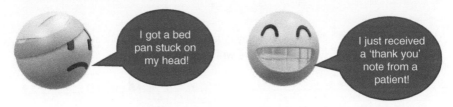

I got a bed pan stuck on my head!

I just received a 'thank you' note from a patient!

It was Patricia Benner who first suggested in 1984 that critical incidents could assist the development of expertise in nursing. She believed that by observing our practice, we can identify any effective or ineffective practice for the task we are undertaking. The words 'critical' and 'incident' can make us think that we are talking about a major event, and possibly in the negative (i.e. that something major has happened). We should, however, be thinking of changing our mindsets to consider them 'learning events', instead. We take learning from both negative and positive events, i.e. when things are going well, as well as when things have gone wrong: This is all part of the learning process, as learning in practice is a continuous process.

HOW IS CRITICAL REFLECTION DIFFERENT TO DESCRIPTION OR REFLECTION?

Critical reflection can be said to be 'careful thinking'. Here are examples of description, reflection, and critical reflection:

Question	Critical reflection, description, or reflection?
What happened?	Descriptive pieces will give an account of scenarios in context. They describe who was involved and their feelings.
Why did this happen? What are the consequences and learning points?	Reflective pieces will build on descriptions to analyse and unfold the account further.
How does this reflect and affect my own practice?	Critical reflection pieces will assess your own capabilities (knowledge and skills) and further learning needs/support.

Mistakes to Avoid when Critically Reflecting

The mistakes to avoid when critically reflecting are these:

- Avoid setting the scene using lengthy descriptions of the scenarios.
- Avoid complaining.
- Avoid blaming (whether yourself, others, or wider circumstances).
- Avoid being too emotional and non-critical.
- Avoid being too objective and scholarly – this is still a personal account.
- Avoid simple problem-solving – there needs to be evidence of personal self-reflection.

CRITICAL REFLECTION MODELS

There are many models for reflecting in practice (see Chapter 3). You may feel that none of these models represents the right model to use in order to 'critically reflect'. It really is a case of what works for you in any given situation/event – it is more about how you **use the model**. Nurses usually use reflective models to guide their practice. This is because placing a structure on this process makes it more purposeful – linking it to the development of critical thinking.

As well as in the healthcare sector, critical reflection is also promoted widely in the social work sector. The Weather Model, which was developed by Maclean (2016) and is used by social workers, can also be used by nurses. This model invites the reflector to reflect on an event or experience using four stages:

	Sunshine	What went well?
	Rain	What didn't go well?
	Lightning	What came as a shock or surprise?
	Fog	What didn't you understand?

Source: Adapted from Maclean (2016).

Following is an example of the Weather Model of reflection, showing that any model of reflection can be adapted to critically reflect on a situation. Honesty is a nursing associate student and is working with Jessica, a newly qualified nursing associate. Patient X has asked for some 'pain killers' as 'that physio terrorist' has put her 'through the wringer'! Honesty looks at the prescription chart and sees that acetaminophen (paracetamol) has been prescribed 'IV or O' – meaning by intravenous or oral route. Even though Honesty knows that Patient X has no swallowing difficulties, she asks Jessica to draw up IV acetaminophen.

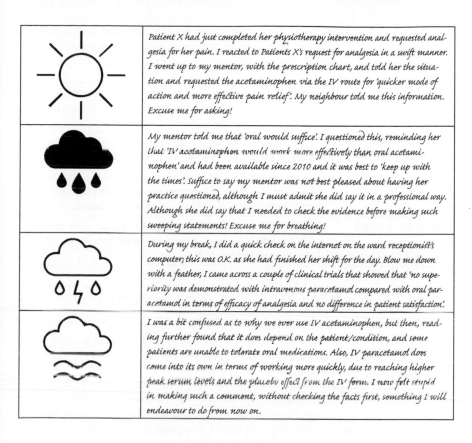

☀	Patient X had just completed her physiotherapy intervention and requested analgesia for her pain. I reacted to Patients X's request for analgesia in a swift manner. I went up to my mentor, with the prescription chart, and told her the situation and requested the acetaminophen via the IV route for 'quicker mode of action and more effective pain relief'. My neighbour told me this information. Excuse me for asking!
🌧	My mentor told me that 'oral would suffice'. I questioned this, reminding her that 'IV acetaminophen would work more effectively than oral acetaminophen' and had been available since 2010 and it was best to 'keep up with the times'. Suffice to say my mentor was not best pleased about having her practice questioned, although I must admit she did say it in a professional way. Although she did say that I needed to check the evidence before making such sweeping statements! Excuse me for breathing!
⛈	During my break, I did a quick check on the internet on the ward receptionist's computer; this was O.K. as she had finished her shift for the day. Blow me down with a feather, I came across a couple of clinical trials that showed that 'no superiority was demonstrated with intravenous paracetamol compared with oral paracetamol in terms of efficacy of analgesia and no difference in patient satisfaction'.
🌫	I was a bit confused as to why we ever use IV acetaminophen, but then, reading further found that it does depend on the patient/condition, and some patients are unable to tolerate oral medications. Also, IV paracetamol does come into its own in terms of working more quickly, due to reaching higher peak serum levels and the placebo effect from the IV form. I now felt stupid in making such a comment, without checking the facts first, something I will endeavour to do from now on.

Honesty has attempted to critically reflect on her practice, acknowledging and questioning practice, but has used some flowery flourishes that may be a little too personal: for example, did we really need to know that she could be blown down with a feather?

Whether we are novices to the practice of critical reflection or more experienced practitioners, we need to critically reflect on the evidence base of our actions to provide good-quality patient care and identify any learning needs we may have. Honesty's neighbour may not be the best source of evidence! An important part of developing our practice at any stage is examining the sources of evidence used when planning patient care and making decisions.

Honesty has started to use the process of critical thinking, whereby evidence is obtained to answer the question 'Am I right'? Sources of evidence may be as follows:

Objective and subjective data	What you have found out through communication, what you observe, what you felt, practice policies and protocols, theoretical ideas.
Communication and observation	The evidence gathered can confirm whether your interpretation was correct or identified deficits.
Assessment of alternatives	Decision-making may have been based on an assessment of the alternatives and possible consequences or on intuition about what you had read or heard.
Feedback of others	Knowing that you made the right decision may come from the feedback of others and what you observed the consequences to be.

WHAT IS CRITICAL THINKING?

Critical reflection involves a degree of critical thinking. To understand the term 'critical thinking', we first need to understand how it differs from 'everyday thinking'. To do this, I will give you an example.

Suppose you and some friends have gone to the local supermarket to buy food for the next couple of days. As it is your birthday tomorrow, and you are all working, your friends have said that they would like to buy you a birthday cake and have asked you to choose which one to buy.

Choice 1 is a large, three-tiered cake with high sugar content.

Choice 2 is a carrot cake with reduced sugar content.

Everyday thinking versus critical thinking:

Everyday thinking	Critical thinking
Choice 1: Yummy – plenty of cake in my tummy! Choice 2: Vegetables in a cake – are you joking? Do I look like a rabbit?	Choice 1: Too much sugar is bad for you. Obesity is a major problem in the UK. Choice 2: This cake may not look as spectacular as the first cake, but it is the healthier choice.
Decision: Cake 1	Decision: Cake 2

You can see that the choice of cake 1 is not objective. Choosing cake 2 is a very simplified version of critical thinking, as it involves applying evidence-based knowledge to your thought processes in coming to a sound conclusion.

STUDENT TIP

Critical thinking is not the same as wondering or guessing.

DEFINING CRITICAL THINKING

There are many definitions of 'critical thinking', but basically it relates to a wide range of intellectual skills that enable individuals to attain expert knowledge as well as apply evidence-based knowledge to new situations in order to come to sound conclusions. In academic work, an important aspect of being critical is distinguishing what is proven and defensible, and combining this with careful speculation. Here is what we can gain in the process of critical thinking:

* Consider a wide variety of viewpoints
* Analyse concepts, theories, and explanations
* Clarify issues
* Examine assumptions
* Assess alleged facts
* Explore implications and consequences
* Think our way to conclusions
* Defend our thinking

- Solve problems
- Transfer ideas to new contexts
- Accept contradictions and inconsistencies in thoughts and experiences

FEATURES OF A CRITICAL THINKER

To be identified as a critical thinker, you need to demonstrate the following features:

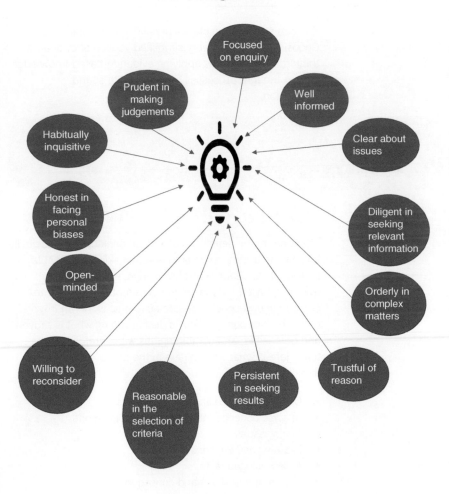

THE STAIRWAY TO CRITICAL THINKING

Williams et al. (2020) devised the critical stairway to critical thinking, whereby to be critical, you step up from description (see Figure 7.1). Following this critical stairway involves the qualities your tutor or instructor is looking for in your work/assignments – these are the qualities that will attract higher grades:

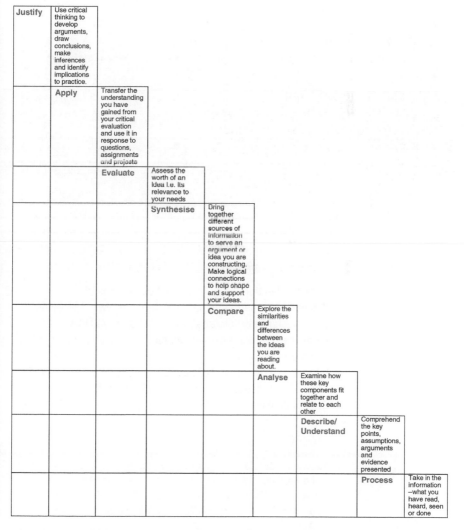

Justify	Use critical thinking to develop arguments, draw conclusions, make inferences and identify implications to practice.						
	Apply	Transfer the understanding you have gained from your critical evaluation and use it in response to questions, assignments and projects					
		Evaluate	Assess the worth of an idea i.e. its relevance to your needs				
			Synthesise	Bring together different sources of information to serve an argument or idea you are constructing. Make logical connections to help shape and support your ideas.			
				Compare	Explore the similarities and differences between the ideas you are reading about.		
					Analyse	Examine how these key components fit together and relate to each other	
						Describe/ Understand	Comprehend the key points, assumptions, arguments and evidence presented
							Process	Take in the information –what you have read, heard, seen or done

Figure 7.1 The critical stairway. Source: Adapted from Williams et al. (2020).

TEST YOUR KNOWLEDGE

Think of an incident in your working life, and document it using the Weather Model of reflection.

KEY POINTS

- What is critical reflection?
- Critical incidents
- How critical reflection differs from description or reflection
- Mistakes to avoid when critically reflecting
- Critical reflection models
- The Weather Model of reflection
- Sources of evidence in reflection
- What is critical thinking?
- Defining critical thinking
- Features of a critical thinker
- The stairway to critical thinking

USEFUL WEB RESOURCES

Critical reflection: https://www.nshcs.hee.nhs.uk
'Benner and expertise in nursing': https://www.sciencedirect.com/science/article/abs/pii/0020748995000113
Intravenous or oral acetaminophen: https://pubmed.ncbi.nlm.nih.gov/29247042/
https://www.cmijournal.org https://emj.bmj.com/content/35/3/179
https://trialbulletin.com/lib/entry/ct-02643394
Critical thinking: https://www.mdpi.com/2079-3200/9/2/22#

RESOURCES

Maclean, S (2016) A new model for social work reflection: whatever the weather. Professional Social Work, March, pp28–29

Williams, K., Woolliams, M., and Spiro, J. (2020). *Reflective Writing: Pocket Study Skills*, 2e. London: Macmillan Education Limited.

Chapter 8
· · · · · · · · · · · · · · · · · · · ·
REFLECTIVE ASSIGNMENTS

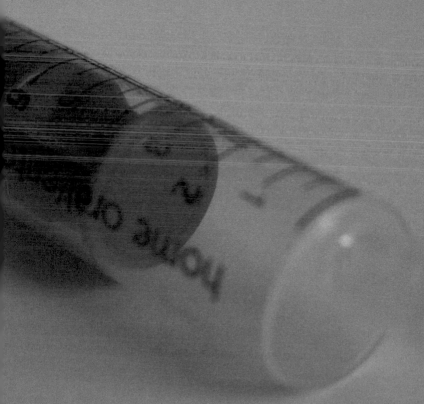

Reflective Practice for Nurses, First Edition. Claire Boyd.
© 2023 John Wiley & Sons Ltd. Published 2023 by John Wiley & Sons Ltd.

LEARNING OUTCOMES

By the end of this chapter, you should have a working knowledge of how to plan and prepare to write an academic reflective essay.

In Chapter 5, we looked at reflective writing, looking at how to use the models of reflection for our **revalidation** (qualified nurses/midwives) or **portfolios** (qualified nurses/midwives and students), or for our **personal use**. We looked at the differences between reports, essays, and reflective writing. You now have an understanding of the reflection process (unless, of course, you skipped those chapters)!

When we reflect by writing for our own personal benefit, we may not necessarily abide by all the academic rules of writing, such as spelling, grammar, sentence construction, paragraphs, etc. However, we do still need to reflect deeply, analytically, and critically on our experience.

We may also be asked to produce an academic reflective assignment. Some of us have difficulty writing academically from a more personal standpoint and in the first person. If that includes you, don't worry; you are not alone: This chapter wasn't originally intended to be included in this book, but when I talked to student nurses, they requested information on writing academic reflective assignments. Your wish is my command!

WHAT SORT OF WRITER ARE YOU?

Before you start to plan your assignment, it is helpful to know what sort of writer you are. This does not need to change when writing formal academic assignments or reflective assignments.

The diver writer	The diver leaps straight in and starts the writing process early on to find out what they want to say. The diver likes to see what emerges before working towards a plan.
The patchwork writer	The patchwork writer works on sections (perhaps using headings) quite early in the process, combining them with linking ideas and words later.
The grand plan writer	The grand plan writer reads and makes notes and leaves writing a plan or beginning the writing process until they have an almost complete picture of the essay ready in their head.
The architect writer	The architect writer has a sense of the structure (perhaps before the content) and may produce a complex plan or spider diagram early in the process.

Source: Adapted from Crème and Lee (1997).

We will now look at how to write reflectively for an academic assignment, starting with the preparation process.

Preparation

When planning to write any assignment, you must first prepare a plan of action, which takes up 9% of the 'writing an assignment' process:

Activity	Percentage of process	What I need to do
Preparing, thinking, and planning	9%	Spend time reading the assignment brief to gain an understanding of what is required.
Searching, reading, and note taking	36%	This is a crucial stage and can be very lengthy. It is important to have a good strategy when searching for the information you need and to keep focused. Use the CRAAP method.
Writing	43%	This is the main part of your plan. You may need to write, rewrite, and rewrite until you are satisfied with your assignment.
Reviewing, editing, proofreading, and final checks	12%	This is the final phase. You should allow yourself plenty of time for this stage. Never skip this stage before you submit your assignment.

DID YOU KNOW?

CRAAP method: Information to assist you when writing an assignment is all around you, but finding good information can be much more difficult. An evaluation tool you can use when you come across information from your literature search is the CRAAP method. Ask these five questions when reviewing information.

Currency: When was the information created?

Relevance: Is the information related to your search?

Accuracy: Is the information factual?

Authority: Who created the information? Has it been peer reviewed?

Purpose: Why was the information created (to inform, teach, sell, etc.)?

MARKING CRITERIA

When writing a formal reflection assignment, you will need to read the marking criteria very carefully. Here are some examples of marking criteria and how the marks are made up. You can see that putting most of your focus on 'correct referencing' (which carries 5 marks) and very little emphasis on 'is it critical and analytical' (which carries 25 marks) will lose you marks and could be the difference between a pass and a referral:

Criteria	Marks available
Explicitly applies a reflective model or framework	10
Includes a clear, detailed, and appropriate description of the experience being reflected on	15
Demonstrates self-awareness Relates relevant theories, concepts, and strategies to nursing practice	15

Criteria	Marks available
Is well presented	5
Is critical and analytical	25
Supports views discussed with evidence	15
Uses correct referencing	5
Effective written communication	10
TOTAL	100

An example of a title for a reflective essay may be 'Reflect on and analyse a critical incident that occurred in clinical practice'. As we already know, this essay will be written in the first person, and the assessor will be looking for evidence of personal and professional growth.

UNDERSTANDING THE QUESTION: PROCESS THE WORDS

When reading through the marking criteria, it is important to understand what the question is actually asking you to do. Following is a brief description of these 'process words', to aid your understanding:

Phrase or word	What it means
Account for	Explain why something happens, clarify, give reasons for.
Analyse	Identify the main points and significant features. Examine critically and/or in great detail.
Assess	Identify the value of, weigh up (see also 'evaluate').
Comment on	Identify the main issues, providing reactions and evidence (examples, sources, authors) to support your points. Avoid personal opinions lacking supporting evidence.
Compare	Show similarities between two (or more) things. Indicate relevance, importance, and consequence of these similarities.
Contrast	Show differences between two (or more) things. Indicate relevance, importance, and consequence of these differences. If appropriate, justify why one item/argument may be more convincing or preferred.

Phrase or word	What it means
Compare and contrast	Show the similarities and differences between two (or more) things.
Criticise	Make a judgement – based on and using examples, evidence, and reasoning – about the merit of two or more related things: for example, theories, opinions, models, items.
Critically evaluate	Weigh arguments for and against something, indicating and then assessing the strength of the evidence on both sides. Be clear about your criteria for how you judge which side is preferable/more convincing.
Define	Provide the exact meaning or a word, concept, or phrase. Where appropriate, you may need to identify other alternative definitions and/or disagreements about the definition.
Describe	Give the main characteristics or features of something, or give a detailed account of it.
Discuss	Explain and give arguments for and against an issue; consider the implications of. Provide evidence to support your points. Often used in connection with a quotation or statement that can be disputed.
Distinguish or differentiate	Look for differences between . . .
Evaluate	Assess the worth, importance, validity, or effectiveness of something using evidence. There will probably be a case both for and against (see 'assess')
Examine	Look in detail – this may also involve 'critical evaluation'
Explain	Clearly identify why something happens or why it is the way that it is.
How far . . .	Usually involves looking at evidence/arguments for and against and weighing them up (see also 'to what extent').
Illustrate	Make clear and explicit, usually requiring carefully chosen examples.
Interpret	Give the meaning and relevance of data or other material.
Justify	Provide evidence supporting an argument/point of view/idea. Show why a decision or conclusions are made, considering and exploring objections.
Narrate	Focus on what happened as a series of events.
Outline	Give only the main features or points on a topic, omitting minor details and emphasising the main structure (see 'summarise')

Phrase or word	What it means
Reflect	Think deeply or carefully about.
Relate	Show similarities and connections between two or more things.
State	Give the main features in a brief and clear form.
Summarise	Draw out the main points only (See 'outline').
Synthesis	Combine information and ideas from multiple sources to develop and strengthen the argument(s).
To what extent . . .	Consider how far something is true and how convincing the evidence is, including any ways in which the opposition remains unproven (see also 'how far . . .').
Trace	Follow the order of different stages in an event or process.

Source: Adapted from Cottrell (2013).

STUDENT TIP

As part of the preparation process, you should also have an awareness of presentation style, font, line spacing, word count, marking criteria, etc. In short, read the brief in full.

Types of Planning: Spider Diagrams/Mind Mapping, Lists

In Chapter 4, we looked at how mind maps (some people refer to them as 'spider diagrams') can be useful in providing a structured way to capture ideas and information, so they can be very useful in planning an assignment and organising your ideas. You use them by starting with an idea and plotting it in the centre of a sheet of paper; this can be the title of the assignment after the topic you have been asked to or have chosen to write about. Then think about ideas you want to include in the essay and how they connect. You may begin by adding a percentage of the word count for the introduction and conclusion as a starting point before adding in the topics you wish to cover in your assignment. For example, here is a mind map for an assignment to write a reflective account of developing leadership styles:

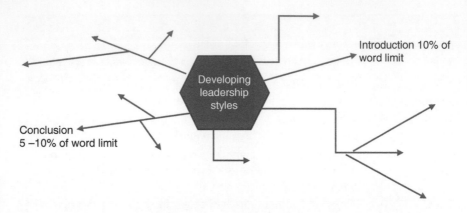

Introduction 10% of word limit

Developing leadership styles

Conclusion 5 –10% of word limit

After you have planned the structure of your essay, you can begin writing. As your nursing career starts, as a pre-graduation (pre-grad) student, your reflective assignments may ask you to analyse and reflect on a specific event in clinical practice using a model of reflection; this may be an example of good or poor practice. For example, you may have observed a poor handover and cite the implications of this in clinical practice.

As your career progresses, and after qualification, you may undertake post-graduation (post-grad) modules, one of which may be to become a manager, as you go up the banding scale. Such a post-grad module may ask you to **reflect on your leadership style** in clinical practice, without the formal structure of a reflective model but using the reflective process of experience, description, analysis, interpretation, perspective, and actions. The following assignment (adaptation) was written some years ago, at level 3, but still applies in showing reflection in action and how the reflective process is used throughout nursing.

AN EXAMPLE OF A REFLECTIVE ASSIGNMENT – LEVEL 3

Understanding Leadership

I presently work for North Bristol NHS Trust (NBT). My present role is as a teacher delivering predominantly clinical skills training, such as male catheterisation, to both professional (e.g. Registered General Nurses and Midwives, and Medics) and non-professional (e.g. Support Workers) under the ethos of the NBT Standard:

'We aim to deliver exceptional healthcare for all our patients, carers and visitors to ensure our care is of the highest quality and our patients are treated with respect and dignity'. (NBT homepage 2016)

I see my role within the NBT Standard to deliver high quality, robust training to staff in order for them to perform clinical skills in a safe and efficient manner and to relay my own teaching experience, skills, and tips to more junior members of the clinical skills team and to lead on their professional development.

Presently I am mentoring a new member of staff within the Staff Development Department in my team. This assignment will focus on my leadership styles and behaviours in relation to my training of this new member of staff in his teaching skills, leading on his professional development plan, and leading the departmental administrative staff in order to support the clinical skills team; thereby taking the form of a work-based approach.

Understand leadership styles

In order to guide my colleague in the teaching of the core clinical skills (such as male catheterisation, etc.), lead on his professional development and, lead the Staff Development support staff, I need to consider three important factors:

- Organisational considerations – how the approach of my leadership style will affect the NBT. Each organisation has its own culture and any change may not be easy to implement. Leading staff in change needs to be managed in a safe and careful manner.
- National considerations – how the approach of my leadership style will affect my colleagues' teaching of the core clinical skills and the implications of this at a National level, i.e. compliance to national strategies and audits.
- Personal considerations – how to match my leadership style appropriately to the task in hand and to my team's preferred leadership style.

The teaching of all the clinical skills needs to be conducted in a consistent and uniform manner, with the strict constraints of following NBT policies and procedures. In short, my colleague has very little room for manoeuvre, following the PowerPoint presentation (which I prepared) almost by the letter in order for the Participants to be aware of how to perform the clinical skill without breaking vicarious liability (Explanation of Vicarious Liability. Figure 1):

Figure 1

Vicarious Liability

Principle by which a practitioner's employer will take liability for the actions and omissions of the employee as long as they are acting within their job description and boundaries approved by the employer.

With this in mind, a *Transactional leadership style* would seem to be appropriate, in that to relay the important information, without any deviation, a task-orientated, structural approach should be initiated when mentoring my colleague in teaching the clinical skills. If this approach is not adhered to, and vital information is not conveyed, this could have cost implications for the organisation. For example, if I had taken a more **Laissez-Faire leadership style** of non-interference, watching from aside, and my colleague had not discussed any infection control issues in core clinical skills subjects, and learners had not been alerted to these risks, infection rates could increase substantially, resulting in non-compliance of quality of clinical improvement audit rates, with heavy fines incurred to NBT. The Health Act (2006) Code of Practice states that NHS Organisations must audit key policies and procedures in order to decrease infection rates, thereby looking at the 'bigger picture' and not just the teaching quality and information relayed. In the case of catheterisation training, as catheter-associated urinary tract infections (CAUTIs) cost an extra £2523 to treat, per patient, it is also the personal repercussions of this to the patient which we need to be mindful of, for example, the misery of longer stays in hospital to treat these infections for the individual.

Due to these vital factors, it may be that a more **Autocratic leadership style** approach should be initiated – which may be the more appropriate leadership style in this case. In short, an approach of 'this is how this needs to be taught and this is what I want taught'. This is a very restrictive and controlling style, but one which is more likely to cover all the key points I want covered, and as the mentor, the preferred leadership style in this case.

The Autocratic leadership style is therefore very much about 'I am the decision maker of what is important and what is not and I will make this decision unilaterally'.

The **Autocratic leadership style** can be viewed in practice during resuscitation situations, as any deviation of the recognised practice of 2 breaths to 30 chest compressions, 100–120 beats per minute, could have life-threatening repercussions on the patient. Therefore, in emergency situations, this style could be viewed as the best leadership style as shouts of 'faster!' enable the health carer to perform the correct technique. In these situations, the leader has to orchestrate the team in a very authoritarian and smooth efficacious manner.

However, different leadership styles fit different situations. Rowe (2007) discusses the fact that being a good leader makes followers want to achieve high goals rather than simply ordering people around – this is known as **emergent leadership**, by **influencing** people rather than **telling them**. Appendix 1 shows two case studies whereby the leadership style required modification to fit the situation.

It should also be noted that Leader and Learner may favour different leadership styles which could cause conflict within teams. In this case it is important to put personality differences to one side and focus on the objectives of the task in hand in order to promote a sense of unity and motivation within the team – known as the **Collegiate leadership style**. It is also important to know who you are leading, as individuals of the team have their own preferred leadership style, and their own strengths and weaknesses, which a good leader can tap into.

Choosing the correct leadership style whilst directing my colleague in the teaching of the core clinical skills could have a negative effect on him. This is due to my preferred perceived leadership style of Autocratic, in teaching situations, which may make him feel he is unable to 'make the session his own' whilst he flexes his teaching muscles. This approach can be quite stifling and disempowering. But not getting the message across could have a very negative effect on the learner and the patient, as discussed previously (due to increased infection rates, etc..).

Keeping control of the session would mean that I could interject throughout, keeping the session on track in relation to getting all the vital points across to the learners. This was a particular concern as my colleague had a tendency to skip over the infection control slides during the presentation, deeming them not important in his opinion.

Interrupting continuously could have a 'belittling' effect on my colleague, with him constantly being interrupted during his session, in front of the learners (something a leader using the Autocratic approach in the classroom situation needs to be mindful of), as well as a disjointed and less enjoyable session for the learners.

However, having talked to him about this, he did express his relief of having the session planned for him via lesson plan, like 'an idiots guide' as his main concern was that he 'would miss something vital'.

He also asked to be interrupted if he 'went off-track' with his teaching. This would seem to indicate that my Autocratic approach was a positive experience for my colleague. As for the group of learners, their evaluation forms from the observed sessions often had comments such as 'trainers very knowledgeable', 'enjoyed the session', and 'learnt a lot', a positive re-enforcement that the Autocratic leadership style did not impact negatively on the training, and in fact the group of learners had benefitted from this leadership style of their trainer.

The Autocratic approach would also be a good style to observe and use himself, when managing new trainers to the Staff Development Department. This is due to the fact that the Department of Health review of operational productivity in the NHS interim report (2016) states that the NHS is presently short of 50 000 staff, equating to a 6% vacancy rate. This could potentially mean more staff to train and extra training staff required.

Understand Leadership Qualities and Review Own Leadership Qualities and Potential

Newstrom & Davis (1993) state that there are four key factors of leadership:

- Know Yourself
- Know human nature
- Know your job
- Know your organisation

Therefore to 'know myself' and in order to reinforce my belief that my Leadership style was indeed 'Autocratic' for the purpose of managing my colleague's teaching session in the core clinical skills, a decision was made to conduct a self-assessment. This self-assessment would take the form of using The Tannenbaum and Schmidt Leadership Continuum questionnaire. I would also conduct the McGregor X and Y Theory, as X and Y leadership styles are at the two furthest ends of the spectrum, enabling me to establish the degree of authority and the degree of autonomy I exercise in my leadership styles.

To my astonishment, according to the Tannenbaum and Schmidt Leadership Continuum tool, I was viewed as being equally weighted between Autocratic and Laissez-Faire leadership styles. I had however noted (as discussed previously) that 'one style does not fit all' as often the leadership style has to be modified to fit the situation. This meant that in practice an Autocratic style would suit certain situations and a different style in other situations, even conducting a modification of many styles in some circumstances.

My colleague completed the same questionnaire and also assessed my leadership styles as equally weighted between a Laisse-Faire and Autocratic. Conducting this exercise did emphasise the fact, such as discussed by Heller (1999) that effective leadership uses elements of each style simultaneously. I had noticed that as my colleague's teaching had improved, in other sessions, I had taken on a less Autocratic style. Marrin (2011) also states that leadership style could be adjusted according to the behaviour and speech according to the situation and audience. In other words, as the person develops, the reins can be loosened and another style can be implemented. However, during a resuscitation incident it could be argued that a confident leader is always required to lead the team and in an Autocratic style.

The U.S. Army (1983) advocate that, as an effective leader, you need to 'know yourself' and 'seek self-improvement'. With this in mind, actions have been developed to enhance my own leadership behaviour in the predominant style of Autocratic. These have been developed from reflecting on my own leadership areas for development, using the SMART approach (Specific, Measureable, Achievable, Relevant, Time based) (Appendix 2).

The actions would be achieved by the end of May, after three months, with a review date of September, 2000 – an achievable time-span and due to my mentee rotating to another department at this time.

This assignment has helped me to develop knowledge and understanding of the Autocratic leadership style and the strengths and weaknesses of using this style in my workplace. It has further shown me that leadership styles are not static and can be adjusted to suit the situation and/or learner

APPENDIX 1

EXAMPLES OF ADAPTING THE LEADERSHIP STYLE TO FIT THE SITUATION

Using the Laisse-Faire Leadership Style

e.g.
EXAMPLE

When interacting with the Staff Development Administrators (training support) I often use the Laisse-Faire leadership style when requesting handouts for training events, stating 'no rush' when in actual fact they are required within a matter of days. This is in order not to put excess pressure on their already heavy workloads. This often results in myself producing a bundle of handouts in case the ordered handouts are not received back from the print room in time. As costs for the departmental printing come out of the Staff Development budget, this has repercussions on the already considerable department overspend and often results in a shortage of paper within the department. Heller (1999) refers to this as having 'difficult conversations' when leading. Using the Laisse-Faire leadership style is therefore not the appropriate leadership style in this case.

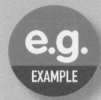

Using the Autocratic Leadership Style

One of the objectives during my colleague's appraisal was to take on a more active role in managing situations. An organisation target and training needs analyst for NBT required a specific ward to receive tracheostomy patients. My colleague was tasked with liaising with the supervisory sisters, in the receiving ward, to establish their staff training requirements. My colleague expressed a lack of confidence in undertaking this task due to 'feeling awkward liaising with higher grade staff than himself'. In this case a more Transformational Leader style was implemented, leading him gently and fully informing him of the organisational requirements and patient safety needs. An Autocratic leadership style would not have worked in this situation.

APPENDIX 2

ACTIONS TO ENHANCE OWN LEADERSHIP BEHAVIOUR

Action	Example	How this will be achieved	When this will be achieved	Review
Action 1 Have an understanding of how the Autocratic leadership style could negatively impact on a person	'Jumping in' during my colleague's teaching session to correct my colleague could have a belittling effect on him, which is not conducive to raising his teaching skills or confidence.	Giving my colleague an in-depth brief about what needs to be relayed during the teaching session, prior to the session.	End of May, 2000	End of September, 2000
Action 2 Learn how to modify the leadership style to fit the situation/ person	The Autocratic leadership style may not always be appropriate when managing my colleagues in every situation.	Conducting an in-depth literature search and reading about leadership styles to increase my knowledge. Learning how to adapt leadership style in different situations, moving along the continuum.	End of May, 2000	End of September, 2000

Action	Example	How this will be achieved	When this will be achieved	Review
Action 3 Be aware of how to communicate effectively	'This is how I do it' is not the same thing as 'This is how I want it done'.	Being crystal clear about standards expected locally (NBT), and Nationally (DOH). Being clear about objectives, e.g. Teaching sessions and/or NBT organisational needs.	End of May, 2000	End of September, 2000
Action 4 Manage difficult situations effectively	Having difficult conversations, e.g. informing support staff exactly what is needed and by when. Informing colleague of teaching strategies to improve performance.	Not being afraid to challenge poor performance. Being mindful of ability to enthuse/guide my colleague in order to raise standards, rather than simply criticise.	End of May, 2000	End of September, 2000

TEST YOUR KNOWLEDGE

1 What are the traits of a 'grand plan' writer?
2 What are the percentages of the process of preparing, thinking, and planning for an assignment?
3 What are the components of the CRAAP literature search?
4 What does the process word 'analyse' mean?
5 What does the process word 'compare' mean?
6 What does the process word 'contrast' mean?
7 What does the process word 'criticise' mean?
8 What does the process word 'critically evaluate' mean?
9 What does the process word 'reflect' mean?
10 What does the process word 'synthesis' mean?

KEY POINTS

- Establishing what sort of writer you are
- Preparing to write your reflective assignment
- CRAAP method of literature search
- Marking criteria – understanding the brief
- Understanding the process words
- Types of planning
- An example of a level 3 assignment, writing in the reflective style

USEFUL WEB RESOURCES

Reflective writing: https://intranet.birmingham.ac.uk/as/
libraryservices/library/asc/documents/public/short-Guide-
Reflective-Writing.pdf

REFERENCES

Crème, P. and Lea, M. (1997). *Writing at University: A Guide for Students*. Buckingham: Open University Press.

Cottrell, S. (2013). *The Study Skills Handbook*, 4e. Basingstoke: Palgrave Macmillan.

Heller, R. (1999). *Effective Leadership*. London: Dorling Kindersley Limited.

Marrin, J. (2011). *Leadership for Dummies*. Ltd. UK: John Wiley & Sons.

Newstrom, J. and Davis, K. (1993). *Organisational Behaviour: Human Behaviour at Work*. New York: McGraw-Hill Publishers.

Rowe, W.G. (2007). *Cases in Leadership*. Thousand Oaks: USA: Sage Publications.

U.S. Army (1983). *Military Leadership. Field Manual 22 – 100*. Washington: DC: U.S. Government Printing Office.

Section Three
· · · · · · · · · · · · · · · · · · · ·
REFLECTION IN PRACTICE

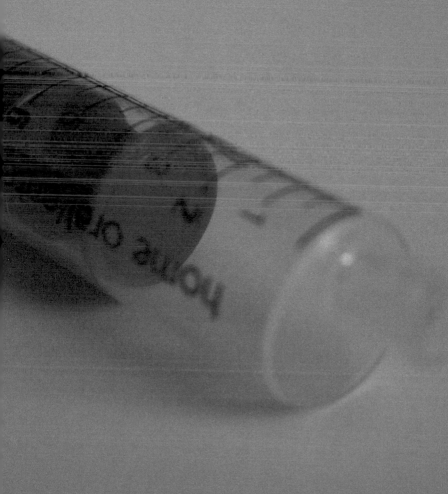

Chapter 9
. . . .
CASE STUDY 1 – NEWLY QUALIFIED NURSE

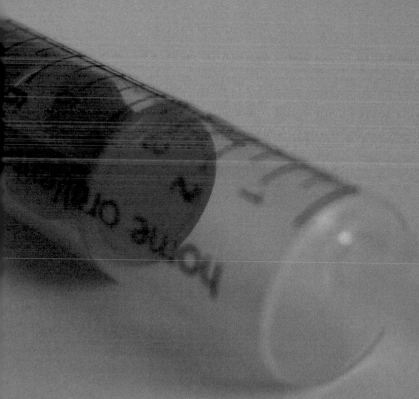

Reflective Practice for Nurses, First Edition, Claire Boyd.
© 2023 John Wiley & Sons Ltd. Published 2023 by John Wiley & Sons Ltd.

LEARNING OUTCOMES

By the end of this chapter, you should have a working knowledge of using Bolton's Through the Looking Glass Model of reflective writing.

NMC HEARINGS AND SANCTIONS

This case study has been adapted from a real-life Fitness to Practice NMC hearing: i.e. a misconduct trial. Only one part of the complaint is discussed here, and there may have been other mitigating aspects to the trial.

USING BOLTON'S THROUGH THE LOOKING GLASS REFLECTIVE WRITING MODEL

Stage	Explanation
Stage 1	Preparation for free writing – letting the content flow with no thought for anything else other than what we want to say on paper.
Stage 2	Free write about the experience we wish to reflect upon – do not worry about grammar, spelling, punctuation or phrasing.
Stage 3	Read our free writing – digest the story we have written
Stage 4	Find someone we trust to read our free writing – ask them to act as our external critical friend. This is called the 'reflective conversation'.
Stage 5	Become reflexive - writing about the same experience from a different point of view. See how our experience impacted those around us to provide us with a different perspective.

Stage	Explanation
Stage 6	After reflecting deeply – prepare our reflective writing for academic purposes (if there is a requirement to do so), going through the content and formatting, shaping and reworking the information into a piece suitable for academic purposes.

Background: Newly qualified nurse put 300 mg of aspirin in a cup to be dispensed, when the prescribed amount was 75 mg.

We can imagine that when reflecting on this drug error, this nurse wrote something like the following:

STAGES 1–2

YESTERDAY

During the early morning drug round, I dispensed patient X's prescribed aspirin into a medicine pot. I was working with Staff Nurse A, who I really don't like, who told me I had made a drug error by putting the wrong dose in the pot. I refuted her observation initially (and was very professional by not asking her to just jog on). She picked up the aspirin pot I had just used and showed me the label, which stated 300 mg aspirin. The patient was prescribed 75 mg of aspirin. We established that there were no pots of 75 mg in the trolley. To be honest, I really don't know what it had to do with her – perhaps she should have been looking after her own patients and minding her own business. It is no wonder I always feel on edge when she is in my vicinity. O.k., so it did become apparent that I had made a mistake, but nothing to get so worked up about – I could just break the tablet into quarters to get the right dose. But apparently this was also the wrong thing to do – give me strength!

I have always known this nurse does not like me and was probably taking satisfaction that I had made a mistake or 'near miss' as she called it. I did feel that she was treating me like a child and this near miss was not such a big deal. Also if my colleagues had not left the drug trolley in a complete mess, then I think the mistake would not have happened, so she had no right just blaming me. I do realise, taking responsibility, that I should have read the drug label on the packaging more closely.

This incident has knocked my confidence and I feel Nurse A could keep this incident just between ourselves as no harm was done. If she reports it, it could affect my career. I have only just finished my preceptorship. I'm beginning to think that my preceptorship was not good enough and this ward needs to review how they conduct this with newly qualified nurses as it is obviously flawed.

I asked Nurse A not to report this incident. I don't really think a dose of 300 mg instead of 75 mg is such a big deal as lots of people take 300 mg of aspirin.

TODAY

After sleeping on it, and reviewing this incident with fresh eyes, I understand why Nurse A could not have kept this incident between ourselves due to the NMC Code, so Nurse A could not just ignore what she had observed.

Our ward Sister told me that it is important not to assume that this drug error could not have caused a great deal of harm to the patient, due to his dehydration and malfunctioning kidneys. After having this discussion with her, and being given information about the harms of aspirin, I now more fully understand the full implications of this incident. I will ask Nurse B, who I have a good relationship with, and I trust, to read through this reflective writing for me for a reflective discussion.

STAGE 3 – Read Out Free Writing

STAGE 4 – Reflective Conversation with Nurse B

STAGE 5

Yesterday I made a drug error, in this case a 'near miss', by dispensing 300 mg of aspirin instead of the prescribed amount of 75 mg. I did not notice I had made this mistake, until it was drawn to my attention. I am now aware how dangerous this could have been to this specific patient. I did at first think that this nurse could have ignored the fact that this mistake had happened, but quickly realised that as nurses, midwives, and nursing associates, we all need to abide by the NMC code.

I feel upset with myself that I did not check the aspirin container more closely – as I know we all need to fully engage in the process of drug administration, and avoid distractions, to avoid making drug errors.

This situation is all very embarrassing for me, as I have to write a report (as does my colleague working with me on that shift). I am presently suspended whilst an investigation (Root Cause Analysis) is being performed. I do now understand that this process is necessary, as patients do expect healthcare professionals not to cause them harm. I fully expect to go down the capability route, whereby my practice will be under scrutiny, which I feel is a good thing because I think I had become a little too complacent when administering medications to patients: This was not my first drug error.

Learning from this mistake, I will be a better nurse by implementing what I have learned during this incident and applying it to my nursing practice:

- *Being more vigilant whilst administering medications*
- *Not being so quick to blame others for my mistakes*
- *Not asking colleagues to cover for my mistakes*
- *Undertaking a period of clinical supervision (which I fully expect to be for a period of approximately six months) depending on the outcome of the investigation*

KEY POINTS

- Drug administration – vigilance
- Drug error – being open and honest
- NMC code
- Aspirin
- Near miss

USEFUL WEB RESOURCES

NMC, latest hearings and sanctions: https://www.nmc.org.uk/concerns-nurses-midwives/hearings/hearings-sanctions/
NMC code: https://www.nmc.org.uk/standards/code/
Aspirin overdose: https://www.drugs.com/medical-answers/aspirin-overdose-symptoms-diagnosis-emergency-3558001

Chapter 10

. . . .

CASE STUDY 2 – NURSING ASSOCIATE

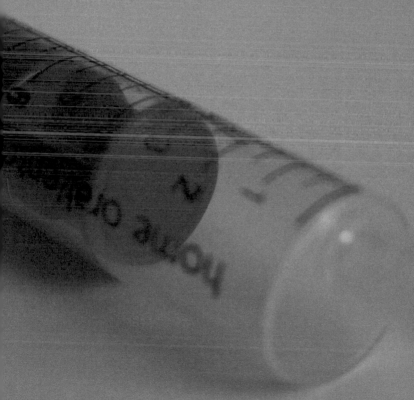

Reflective Practice for Nurses, First Edition, Claire Boyd.
© 2023 John Wiley & Sons Ltd. Published 2023 by John Wiley & Sons Ltd.

LEARNING OUTCOMES

By the end of this chapter, you should have a working knowledge of using experience, reflection, action (ERA) reflection (2013).

NMC HEARINGS AND SANCTIONS

This case study has been adapted from a real-life Fitness to Practice NMC hearing: i.e. a misconduct trial. Only one part of the complaint is discussed here, and there may have been other mitigating aspects to the trial.

USING THE ERA MODEL OF REFLECTION

This model was developed by Jasper in 2013 and is one of the simpler models of reflection. It consists of three steps:

1 Experience – Which can be positive or negative
2 Reflection – Thinking through the experience and examining our feelings after what has happened
3 Action – What we do as a result of the experience, depending on our feelings and experiences leading up to it

TERMINOLOGY

SHO: Senior house officer
PRN: As-required medication (Pro Ra Nata)
Anti-pyretic: Substance that reduces fever
RGN: Registered general nurse
NSAID: Non-steroidal anti-inflammatory drug

Background: Nursing associate dispensed one paracetamol tablet instead of two. Failed to respond to patient having a high temperature.

We can imagine that when reflecting on this drug error, this nurse associate wrote something like the following:

Experience

I am a Nursing Associate and had just performed the clinical observations of a patient, whereby I found his heart rate, respirations, and temperature elevated: HR: 91 = 1, Respirations: 21 = 2, Temperature: 38.1 = 1, generating a combined NEWS II score of 4.

I know that paracetamol has anti-pyretic properties and found that he had been prescribed 500 mg to 1 gram of paracetamol PRN, which he had not yet been administered. I thought, as he was quite elderly, I would administer 1 tablet (500 mg). I contacted the patient's SHO and informed her about his observations 'triggering' and told her I had administered his anti-pyretic medication, as prescribed.

Some time later (4 hours), I went back to his room to take his temperature again and found his heart rate, respirations, and temperature has risen even further: HR: 110 = 1, Respirations: 25 = 3, Temperature: 39.0 = 1, generating a combined NEWS II score of 5. He was slightly delirious, very pale and sweaty. I immediately called his SHO again, after removing one of his blankets from his bed and performing tepid sponging of his skin to cool the patient down.

Reflection

Even though I followed protocol on the NEWS II observation chart by monitoring the patient 'with a score of 1–4, 4–6 hourly', I had forgotten to inform the Nurse-in-charge of the situation initially, whereby it is up to her/him to make the decision whether to increase the frequency of the monitoring. It was also apparent, after the SHO came to assess the patient, that I should have administered 1 gram of the paracetamol, which the SHO assumed I had. Also that I had not administered the ibuprofen (NSAID) prescribed PRN (which I did not know also had anti-pyrexial properties), so should have administered this. I was also informed that tepid sponging should be avoided as I was now told it 'cools the skin' temporarily and can make the condition worse by inducing shivering, which raises the core body temperature.

I do feel like a fool and I should have known these basic principles of temperature control. The very least I could have done was to open the window for ventilation in this very hot room. I do believe that some nursing staff look down on Nursing Associates (not quite realising the full extent of our academic training) and that we are not as good as other members of the healthcare profession with university degrees, and my mistake will add fuel to the fire.

When I was asked to explain my actions, I really don't know why I acted the way I did, which I know is no excuse. To make matters worse, the Nurse-in-charge asked me, earlier on in the shift, as well as a Registered General Nurse working in my team, if everything was O.K. with my patients and I told both of them, everything was 'fine'. I should have told them about this patient and the fact that I had called the SHO to review the patient. I don't think they are very happy with me.

Action

What I have learnt from this situation, if faced with a similar situation, is that I will apply thermal-regulation principles to apyrexial patients, and not undertake tepid bathing on these patients. I will also take forward the information that I must keep the Nurse-in-Charge fully informed and up-to-date about my patients. I have also learnt from the confusion I caused whereby the SHO had assumed that when I said I had administered the anti-pyretic medication, that I had administered 1 gram paracetamol and ibuprofen – I will in future state exact dosages to the SHOs. Although I think she is somewhat to blame for this as well. I will also carry forward the information I have gained about the NEWS II observation chart whereby we do not need to follow the instructions by the letter, as we can use our own professional judgement. In this case conducting more frequent observations in this situation would have been more appropriate.

I am very upset about my mistake and have not stopped crying. My Manager has been very kind and I agree with her that I should get signed off sick, as I am in no fit state to work at present. My Manager has also told me to confide in a trusted colleague, as I will need all the support I can get.

I have made quite a few mistakes in my nursing practice, which I have been alerted to previously, and am working through. I feel this may be the last straw.

KEY POINTS

- ERA Model of Reflection
- The importance of communication within teams
- Thermoregulation principles
- How to use the NEWS II observation chart effectively

USEFUL WEB RESOURCES

NMC, latest hearings and sanctions: https://www.nmc.org.uk/concerns-nurses-midwives/hearings/hearings-sanctions/
Pyrexia: https://www.ncbi.nlm.nih.gov/pmc/articles/pmc5047044

Chapter 11

. . . .

CASE STUDY 3 – MENTAL HEALTH NURSE

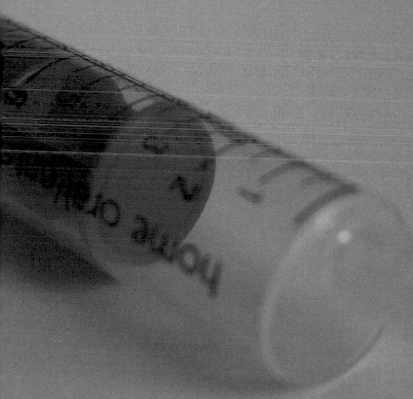

Reflective Practice for Nurses, First Edition. Claire Boyd.

NMC HEARINGS AND SANCTIONS

This case study has been adapted from a real-life Fitness to Practice NMC hearing: i.e. a misconduct trial. Only one part of the complaint is discussed here, and there may have been other mitigating aspects to the trial.

USING THE ROLF ET AL. MODEL OF REFLECTION

What?	Outline the situation (descriptive).
So what?	Discuss what you have learnt (theory and knowledge building).
Now what?	Identify the implications (action oriented).

DID YOU KNOW?

Disulfiram: A drug used to support the treatment of alcohol use disorder by producing an acute sensitivity to ethanol. Disulfiram works by inhibiting the enzyme acetaldehyde dehydrogenase, causing many of the effects of a hangover to be felt immediately following alcohol consumption. Disulfiram plus alcohol – even small amounts – produces flushing, a throbbing headache, respiratory difficulty, nausea, copious vomiting, sweating, thirst, chest pain, palpitation, dyspnoea, hyperventilation, tachycardia, hypotension, fainting, marked uneasiness, weakness, vertigo, blurred vision, and confusion. In severe reactions, there may be respiratory depression, cardiovascular collapse, abnormal heart rhythms, myocardial infarction, acute congestive heart failure, unconsciousness, convulsions, and death.

Drug classes: aldehyde dehydrogenase inhibitor.

Background: Mental health nurse failed to breathalyse a patient prior to administering disulfiram.

We can imagine that when reflecting on this drug error, this nurse wrote something like the following:

What?	I am a Mental Health Nurse and responsible for a patient detained under the Mental Health Act (1983), Section 17 leave; meaning they are detained under the Mental Health Act, but authorised by a responsible Clinician to leave hospital. Patient was due to receive his prescribed dose of Disulfiram medication (and B12 injection), which I duly administered. I had previously been reprimanded by my Manager that morning, for my time management issues ('constantly arriving late for work') and for not following protocol when calling in sick, so my mind was not fully on my work when patient X came into the unit for his appointment, as I was extremely upset about the unfairness of my reprimand.
So what?	After I had just given patient X his prescribed Disulfiram, my Manager came over to where I was working and started giving me a right rollocking for not breathalysing the patient prior to administering the medication and how dangerous this was. I admitted my mistake as I had, in all honesty, just forgotten to do this. I think I should have been given some credit for admitting this. I told my manager that I had learnt from this and would never make this mistake again (basically get over it – mistakes happen)! There was really no need for my manager to rub salt into the wound by handing me an information sheet about Disulfiram. I found this insulting. The patient getting wind of all this, started complaining that he felt unwell, experiencing 'a throbbing headache and feeling nauseous with chest pain'. I don't believe a word of it, as I think he was just trying to get me into trouble.
Now what?	By this point, I had had enough and told my manager that I felt ill and went home. I feel this was the best option as I was getting angry and stressed. I know the implications of my error, so don't need my nose rubbed in it, and had to think about my own mental health. I will be more vigilant when administering medications in future, so as not to harm patients. End of story!

KEY POINTS

- Mental Health Act (1983)
- Rolf et al. Model of Reflection (2001)
- Disulfiram

USEFUL WEB RESOURCES

NMC, latest hearings and sanctions: https://www.nmc.org.uk/
concerns-nurses-midwives/hearings/hearings-sanctions/

Mental Health Act (1983): https://www.nhs.uk/mental-health/
social-care-and-your-rights/mental-health-and-the-law/
mental-health-act

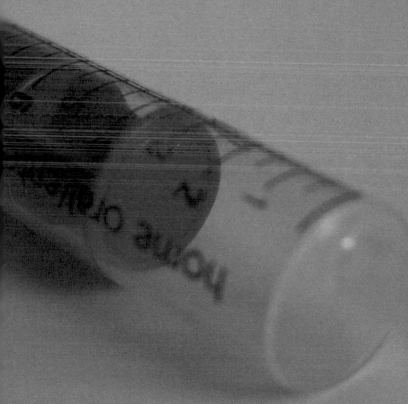

Chapter 12
· · · · · · · · · · · · · · · · · ·
CASE STUDY 4 – QUALIFIED NURSE

LEARNING OUTCOMES

By the end of this chapter, you should have a working knowledge of using the REFLECT Model of reflection.

NMC HEARINGS AND SANCTIONS

This case study has been adapted from a real-life Fitness to Practice NMC hearing: i.e. a misconduct trial. Only one part of the complaint is discussed here, and there may have been other mitigating aspects to the trial.

USING THE REFLECT MODEL OF REFLECTION

Recall the events	Stage 1: Give a brief overview of the situation on which you are reflecting. This should consist of the facts – a description of what happened.
Examine your responses	Stage 2: Discuss your thoughts and actions at the time of the incident on which you are reflecting.
Acknowledge Feelings	Stage 3: Highlight any feelings you experienced at the time of the situation on which you are reflecting.
Learn from the experience	Stage 4: Highlight what you have learnt from the situation.
Explore options	Stage 5: Discuss options for the future if you were to encounter a similar situation.
Create a plan of action	Stage 6: Create a plan for the future – this can be for further theoretical learning or action.
Set a Timescale	Stage 7: Set a time by which the plan outlined in stage 6 will be completed.

Background: Qualified nurse administered Oramorph (morphine sulphate), an oral medication, to patient by incorrect route, namely subcutaneous injection.

We can imagine that when reflecting on this drug error, this nurse wrote something like the following:

Stage 1

I am an experienced Registered Nurse of five years standing and recently started work in a new clinical directorate (6 months ago) due to problems in my last clinical area. Patient RU was prescribed oral Oramorph, which I knew to be Morphine Sulphate. I have administered Morphine Sulphate Subcutaneously (SC), IM, and IV previously to patients. I have never come across an 'oral' format of this drug. I duly drew up the medication in a syringe and administered it to the patient subcutaneously. Sister came running up to me, seeing what I was doing, and told me to stop. Unfortunately, I had completed the injection and was really confused as to what I had done wrong. I was immediately told that I had administered this medication via the wrong route (and did not have a colleague check this controlled drug with me, as per policy).

Stage 2

During my last IV update, we had been told about a patient called Wayne Jowett, who had died due to a wrong route drug administration error, and this tragic mistake had really upset me. I was completely inconsolable about making a similar wrong route drug administration error and started crying. I just wanted to go home and never set foot in the hospital again.

Stage 3

Whilst the Medics and other staff came to sort out the patient, Sister took me into the office and asked why I had given oral Oramorph via the S/C route. I thought it best to be honest and told her that this was due to lack of knowledge/training.

Stage 4

Sister was very kind to me but explained that this was a serious mistake, known as 'a never event' in the NHS and would need to be investigated. Never events are serious incidents that are considered entirely preventable. She also stated that I would need to 'get all my ducks lined up' ready for this investigation. I was told that I would need to go home until further notice and Sister would arrange for another staff member to drive me home, as I was obviously in no fit state to *drive myself home. While I was waiting in the office, I did think that it really was not as bad as Sister had made out as Morphine Sulphate is Morphine Sulphate, so as I was waiting I went on the internet to gather some information and came across a report by The Healthcare Safety Investigation Branch (HSIB) who conduct independent investigations of patients safety concerns in the NHS, about a similar mistake as mine, i.e. the administration of an oral liquid into a vein. It made for traumatic reading, explaining that medicine administered by an incorrect route can cause serious sometimes long lasting effects and can often be fatal for the patient.*

I then went on to look at the differences between oral Morphine Sulphate and injectable Morphine Sulphate and found their ingredients to be somewhat different:

Oral Morphine Sulphate: *Morphine Sulphate, Ethanol (alcohol), sucrose, methylparahydroxybenzoate (E218), and propylparahydroxybenzoate (E216).*

IV/IM Morphine Sulphate: *Morphine Sulphate, sodium chloride, Trisodium citrate dihydrate, edetate disodium, calcium chloride, and water.*

Stage 5

After I had conducted this search on the internet, I now fully realised that the error I had made was a serious one, and I had put this patient at risk. I had learnt the hard way and taking time to think about the ways I would have changed things, I realised that I should not have cut corners and got another staff member to sign out and check the controlled drug with me, as per policy, and this mistake could have been adverted. During this time of reflection, I also realised other implications for the patient from my 'Never Event' – that of patients losing trust in the healthcare system, and prolonged patient hospitalisation producing extra healthcare costs. I also realised that I should know about any medication I administer, and if I don't, to find out. It is no good saying my knowledge was lacking – I needed to do something about this.

Stage 6

I don't yet know what will happen with the investigation, and where this will take me, but I do know I need to take responsibility for my actions. In the meanwhile I will increase my knowledge on drug administration (I have seen a very good book on this which I will buy). Something else I just thought about would be to remember the basic rule of drug administration we were taught all those years ago, and which I know has been extended, i.e. to 10 or 15 Rights: But using the basic Five Rights, which I did not implement today, in other words, always checking before administrating medications:

- *Right Patient*
- *Right Medication*
- *Right Dose*
- *Right Route*
- *Right Time*

Stage 7

When the dust has settled, and if I am to go down the capability route, Sister and I can sit down and prepare an action plan and time scale.

KEY POINTS

- REFLECT Model of reflection
- Oral Oramorph
- Morphine sulphate IM/IV
- Never events
- Wrong route drug administration
- Implications of drug errors
- Controlled drugs policies and procedures
- The Five Rights of drug administration

USEFUL WEB RESOURCES

NMC, latest hearings and sanctions: https://www.nmc.org.uk/concerns-nurses-midwives/hearings/hearings-sanctions/

Morphine: https://www.drugs.com/morphine

NHS, questions about morphine: https://www.nhs.uk/medicines/morphine/common-questions-about-morphine

Medication administration drug errors: https://www.ncbi.nlm.nih.gov/pmc/articles/PMC7764714/

Chapter 13

. . . .

CASE STUDY 5 – LEARNING DISABILITY NURSE

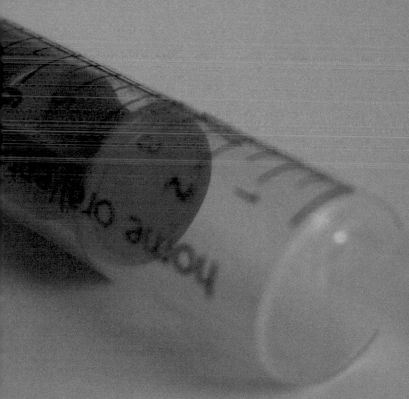

Reflective Practice for Nurses, First Edition. Claire Boyd.

LEARNING OUTCOMES

By the end of this chapter, you should have a working knowledge of the Gibbs Reflective Cycle.

NMC HEARINGS AND SANCTIONS

This case study has been adapted from a real-life Fitness to Practice NMC hearing: i.e. a misconduct trial. Only one part of the complaint is discussed here, and there may have been other mitigating aspects to the trial.

USING THE GIBBS REFLECTIVE CYCLE

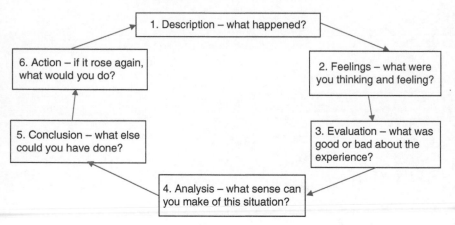

1. Description – what happened?

2. Feelings – what were you thinking and feeling?

3. Evaluation – what was good or bad about the experience?

4. Analysis – what sense can you make of this situation?

5. Conclusion – what else could you have done?

6. Action – if it rose again, what would you do?

Background: Learning disability nurse did not prime a syringe before administering insulin.

We can imagine that when reflecting on this drug error, this nurse wrote something like the following:

1   *I was about to administer insulin to a Service User with constant uncontrolled type 1 diabetes experiencing hyperglycaemia. Medics had been mystified as to why this Service User's blood glucose levels were not stabilising. I was stopped by a colleague who stated that I must not administer this insulin I had just drawn up, as there was a huge air bubble in*

the syringe, meaning that the patient was not getting the correct dosage of the medication, as prescribed.

2   At first, I did not think that the air bubble would make much difference and I did not like having my practice questioned. I do think people can get too wrapped up about tiny little air bubbles in IV lines and syringes. But I did think about this situation and wondered whether it could be true that I was contributing to the patient's hyperglycaemia by not, inadvertently, administering the correct dose of insulin required, due to the air bubble in the syringe, i.e. Service User would not get the dose on the syringe as 2 mLs of the syringe contents were taken up by the air bubble.

3   I did reflect on the situation and as the insulin was to be administered subcutaneously, the air bubble would not have been a problem, as my training had always told me that injecting a small air bubble into the skin or a muscle is usually harmless. I also know that when an air bubble enters a vein, it is called a venous air embolism and when an air bubble enters an artery, it is called an arterial air embolism and can be fatal, as these air bubbles can travel to your brain, heart, or lung and cause a myocardial infarction (heart attack), cerebral vascular accident (stroke), or respiratory failure.

4   I realise that the air bubble is not such an issue; the shortfall of the insulin caused by the air bubble was more the issue. I think my focus was on the wrong thing. Also, what I had considered to be a minor blip initially, such as not receiving the correct dosage of insulin, is much more serious than I had first suspected. I came to this conclusion after conducting a search on the internet and found that long-term hyperglycaemia can lead to serious health problems, if left untreated, such as Diabetic Ketoacidosis (potentially leading to a diabetic coma) and something called Hyperosmolar Hyperglycaemic State (severe dehydration). This Service User regularly has high blood sugar levels, which a further internet search informed me could result in permanent damage to the eyes, nerves, kidneys, and blood vessels. This all made me realise that I had been contributing to this Service User's condition, as he had been in our care for many years and I was his named carer.

5   I now undertook advice, from my work colleague, on how to prime a syringe, removing air bubbles, and this is what I learnt and intend to implement when next drawing up insulin (or any injection):

   a   After preparing the insulin vial and syringe, and checking all the details, hold the vial of insulin down and push the needle of the syringe into the vial. I will need to ensure that the end of the needle of the syringe is in the insulin liquid and not out of the insulin and drawing up air. Draw up the required number of units plus a few units more.

   b   Remove any bubbles by holding the syringe with the needle pointing upwards and tap the syringe with the finger or the tip of the fingernail.

C   *With the syringe still upright, push the plunger into the syringe until the required number of units remain in the syringe. Remove the syringe from the vial. If air is still in the syringe, tap the syringe again to remove.*

6   *Thanks to my colleague and friend, I now know how to prime a syringe and can understand how this impacted on the Service User's blood glucose levels over a considerable time frame. My colleague also helped me to understand what to observe for signs of hyperglycaemia, such as:*

- *Increased thirst and dry mouth (which the Service User experiences)*
- *Needing to pee frequently (which the Service User experiences)*
- *Tiredness (which the Service User experiences)*
- *Blurred vision*
- *Unintentional weight loss*
- *Recurrent infections (such as thrush, bladder infections, and skin infections)*
- *Stomach pains*
- *Nausea and vomiting*
- *Breath that smells of pear drops*

Undertaking this Model of Reflection has enabled me to be a better nurse due to increasing my knowledge on hyperglycaemia. I will practice this new found knowledge for now on.

KEY POINTS

- Using the Gibbs Reflective Cycle
- Hyperglycaemia and the adverse effects on the body
- How to prime a syringe, removing air bubbles
- The dangers of venous and arterial air embolisms

USEFUL WEB RESOURCES

NMC, latest hearings and sanctions: https://www.nmc.org.uk/concerns-nurses-midwives/hearings/hearings-sanctions/

Injections: http://www.peacehealth.org/medical-topics/id/abs5701

Hyperglycaemia: https://www.nhs.uk/conditions/high-blood-sugar-hyperglycaemia

Air embolism: https://www.nhs.uk/conditions/air-embolism/

Chapter 14

· · · · · · · · · · · · · · · · · · · ·

CASE STUDY 6 – MIDWIFE

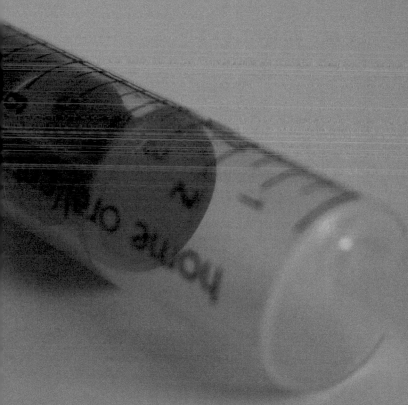

Reflective Practice for Nurses, First Edition. Claire Boyd.

LEARNING OUTCOMES

By the end of this chapter, you should have a working knowledge of the NMC Reflective Account documentation.

NMC HEARINGS AND SANCTIONS

This case study has been adapted from a real-life Fitness to Practice NMC hearing: i.e. a misconduct trial. Only one part of the complaint is discussed here, and there may have been other mitigating aspects to the trial.

USING THE NMC REFLECTIVE ACCOUNT MODEL

Background: Midwife failed to recognise a double-dose prescription error for (acetaminophen) paracetamol.

We can imagine that when reflecting on this drug error, this nurse wrote something like the following:

Reflective Account: Drug Error

What was the nature of the CPD activity and/or practice-related feedback and/or event or experience in your practice?

I had been caring for a primigravida individual and she asked for `something for her headache' due to her `flu'. As she was some way off from her delivery, I consented to her request (after I was unable to dissuade her from taking any medication for the present). After she had taken 1 gram of paracetamol, I remembered that I had previously administered her prescribed co-codamol (for her dentistry problems and prescribed by her GP), which I now remembered also contains paracetamol. To add to my dismay, she also informed me that she had `not long ago' taken an over-the-counter cold and flu remedy, which also contained paracetamol. In short, I had basically administered a double dose of paracetamol.

*I felt terrible and I **immediately** informed the nurse-in-charge and the Medical team and recorded a full set of observations. The team seemed very annoyed with me and I did not feel supported, as I was devastated that I had made this drug error. I was relieved of my duties but told to collect an intravenous bag of `acetylcysteine' first and then to go to the office to write a reflective account before going home.*

What did you learn from the CPD activity and/or feedback and/or event or experience in your practice?

Whilst writing my reflective account, I undertook a Google search about the dangers of paracetamol overdose. An NHS site informed me that adults can take a maximum of four doses in 24 hours and to wait at least 4 hours between doses. My expectant mother had taken a double dose. I read that paracetamol overdoses are the leading cause of liver failure in Britain and usually occur when patients take a vast number of tablets all at once and that a liver transplant may be required if damage to the liver becomes severe (https://www.nhs.uk/medicines/paracetamol-for-adults).

It was at this point I realised the full implications of my mistake, and basically how much trouble I was in. I wanted to apologise to the expectant mother, but the nurse-in-charge did not want me to have any contact with her at present due to her `devastation' and fear that I had `harmed her baby'.

I researched the antidotes to treat paracetamol overdose, which are:

1 *Activated charcoal treatment (administered within first hour of overdosing)*
2 *Intravenous acetylcysteine (treatment can be given up to 24 hours after overdose)*
3 *Oral methionine*

I also viewed graphs for paracetamol toxicity, according to body weight and amount of paracetamol ingested. I believe none of the antidotes had been administered, just regular monitoring of both mother and baby, as the overdose I had administered was not considered life threatening I believe.

How did you change or improve your practice as a result?

*All the information I had gained would enhance my practice, and I know I would never again make this drug error again. I will always follow the Drug Administration Policy and first ask individuals if they have taken any medication that day and '**Before taking any other medicines, check the label to see whether they contain paracetamol**' before I administer it and not after, like I did with the co-codamol.*

I am aware that I will be disciplined for my error as some may consider that as an experienced healthcare professional, I should have known better. Before I leave today, I will contact my Union Representative to seek representation and talk to my colleague and best friend for support, as the more I write about this incident, the more upset I feel (this was the nurse-in-charge's advice to me). I do wonder if some of the other mistakes I have made at work will be used against me.

How is this relevant to the Code?

Preserve Safety:

16: Act without delay if you believe that there is a risk to patient safety or public protection.

18: Advise on, prescribe, supply, dispense, or administer medicines within the limits of your training and competence, the law, our guidance, and other relevant policies, guidance, and regulations.

Promote Professionalism and Trust:

23: Cooperate with all investigations and audits

24: Respond to any complaints made against you professionally

KEY POINTS

- Using the NMC Reflective Account model documentation
- The dangers of acetaminophen (paracetamol) overdose
- Antidotes to acetaminophen toxicity
- The importance of vigilance when administering acetaminophen (for covert acetaminophen in other medications)
- The importance of following policies and procedures

USEFUL WEB RESOURCES

NMC, latest hearings and sanctions: https://www.nmc.org.uk/concerns-nurses-midwives/hearings/hearings-sanctions/

Paracetamol: https://www.nhs.uk/medicines/paracetamol-for-adults

NMC: www.nmc.org.uk/standards/code

Chapter 15

· · · · · · · · · · · · · · · · · · ·

REFLECTION IN PRACTICE – REFLECTIVE JOURNAL EXTRACT

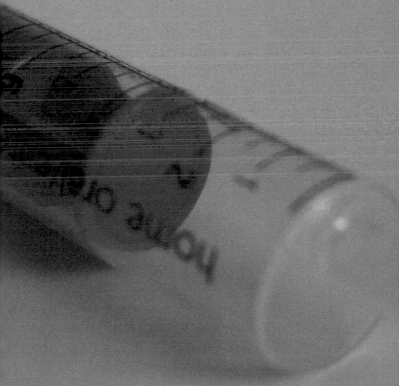

Reflective Practice for Nurses, First Edition. Claire Boyd.
© 2023 John Wiley & Sons Ltd. Published 2023 by John Wiley & Sons Ltd.

LEARNING OUTCOMES

By the end of this chapter, you should have a working knowledge of writing reflectively in a journal and the learning that can be taken from this.

This piece is an adaption of a journal entry written by a newly qualified nurse during the first wave of the Covid-19 pandemic in the UK. It shows how reflection can often be cathartic.

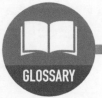

GLOSSARY

Cathartic
Providing a psychological relief through the open expression of strong emotions, causing catharsis.

It also shows the learning taken place in regard to taking the positives from often very bleak situations in practice and how important colleagues can be to lean on to help get you through difficult times. In addition, it shows the life-long learning aspect to reflective journals, whereby what we learn can be carried forward in our nursing career.

This nurse decided to use a framework in her journal:

- Observe
- Discuss
- Analyse
- Reflect

OBSERVE

Yesterday had been yet another shift from hell. It's all getting too much; I am literally just existing – work, eat, sleep, work, eat, sleep. My face has come out in spots due to the restricting PPE and I am just exhausted all the time. This is like a nightmare. I feel so stressed, angry, and depressed. Everyone else seems to be coping better than me, and although I have not told anyone, I am really scared that I will catch Covid and die, or worse take it home to my partner – I think about death and my own mortality all the time now. I came in to nursing as I always thought this was more like a calling than a job, but I really hate this situation. Everything is just so heart-breaking and all I do at home is cry – perhaps I am not really cut out to be a nurse at all. Yesterday we organised a video call for a patient who was on his way out and his family had to say their good-byes over the phone: He had been married for over 20 years and his wife and family couldn't ever hold his hand and be with him. It is all just too much, too heart-breaking and cruel.

DISCUSS

As I was getting ready to go home, one of my colleagues came into the changing rooms crying, which started me off again!. We talked about our exhaustion and heartbreak and how scared we were. We are both demoralised and have lost hope. Our other colleague came into the room and told us that we were all feeling the same, and should talk and debrief, i.e. not carry our feelings alone. She also mentioned that we would get through this together. That got us all talking about recharging our bodies 'between assaults' by resting and eating proper meals and not grabbing bags of crisps and an orange, like we are tending to do, due to being too tired to cook after a shift. She also reminded us of all the patients we had cared for that had got better and the difference we had all made. This made us all think that the negatives have been over-whelming, but there have been many positives.

ANALYSE

I got thinking about what my colleagues and I discussed in the cloak-room and how important it is to talk to colleagues and not to think that you are the only one feeling scared and disheartened. It was good to know that everyone is feeling vulnerable and we are not alone. This made me do a quick Google search to find the importance of communicating with others and looking after our own mental health.

REFLECT

There is an old saying 'a problem shared is a problem halved' – at least I think it is something like this! This has made me realise that we are a team and should not carry our emotions alone, but to share this with others, which is good for our mental health. Sharing our feelings is not a weakness but shows courage. This is something I will carry with me throughout my time as a nurse.

Also, I do think that I had lost sight of the positives: On the way to work today I saw house windows full of pictures of rainbows – thanking the NHS. This made me feel proud and valued, and very emotional. Also, some of us were told to leave our clinical areas and go out at 8 p.m. for a short while to listen to the 'clapping for carers' whereby members of the public clap outside their homes to show their gratitude for the essential workers (health carers, teachers, police and fire services, shop workers, security guards, etc.). This made us feel so appreciated and has been a huge morale booster. I know I will have other difficult shifts in the future, and I am still considering leaving the nursing profession when this terrible time is over, but I will try to remember this feeling to keep me going in the meanwhile. I have also realised the importance of talking to colleagues about our feelings, as this is not a weakness, but important for our mental health. I know this is something I can apply to whatever career choice I may chose in the future.

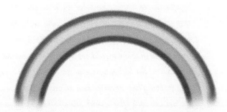

KEY POINTS

- Writing for reflective journals
- The importance of communication within teams
- The importance of looking after your own mental health
- Learning from writing reflective journals

USEFUL WEB RESOURCES

Importance of communication: https://www.calmsage.com/why-communication-is-the-key-to-mental-wellness

Sharing emotions for mental health wellness:
https://www.nih.gov/health-information/emotional-wellness-toolkit
https://goodmenproject.com/health/the-benefits-of-sharing-emotions/

Answers

Activity 1.1

Let's see how self-aware you are.
Complete the Johari window for yourself.

OPEN	BLIND
Known to self and to others	Not known to self but known to others
HIDDEN	**UNKNOWN**
Known to self but not to others	Not known to self or others

ANSWER: This will be personal to you.

Test Your Knowledge

1 What are the 10 essential ingredients for successful reflection?
ANSWER:
- Academic skills
- Knowledge
- Attitudinal qualities
- Self-awareness
- Being person centred
- Being empathic
- Communication
- Mindfulness
- Being process-orientated
- Being strategic

2 What are the two main types of reflection?
ANSWER: Informal and formal

3 What is reflective practice?
ANSWER: Thinking about a situation or experience and learning from it.

Reflective Practice for Nurses, First Edition. Claire Boyd.
© 2023 John Wiley & Sons Ltd. Published 2023 by John Wiley & Sons Ltd.

4 The reflective process should contain six essential elements. What are they?
ANSWER:
- Incident/experience (positive or negative)
- A description
- An analysis
- An interpretation
- A perspective
- An action

5 Name four benefits of reflection in nursing.
ANSWER:
- Enhances patient care delivery
- Critical reflection awareness
- Improves problem-solving skills of the workforce
- Enhances effectiveness of the individual

6 What are the six C's of nursing:
ANSWER:
- Care
- Compassion
- Competence
- Communication
- Courage
- Commitment

7 What do learning journals usually include?
ANSWER:
- A summary of the event
- Facts relating to the incident
- Immediate learning points
- Thoughts/feelings at the time

8 Why do we **need** to reflect in nursing?
ANSWER:
- Professional body requirements
- For the Knowledge and Skills Framework

- Course requirements
- Self-development

CHAPTER 2

Activity 2.1

Take a moment to think about the question 'What makes your working day difficult?
ANSWER: This will be personal to you. Here are the answers some others have come up with:

Personality clash	Poor team dynamics
Challenges	No breaks
Poor culture	Disorganisation
Poor leadership	Not sharing ideas or thoughts
Not all singing from the same song sheet	No thanks
No support/too heavy workload	Hierarchy factors at play
Low morale	Conflict
Not confident	Others taking credit for the work you do
Lazy colleagues	Demotivation
No staff	Poor attitude

Activity 2.2

What do you think are the five most common medications to be implicated in incidents, according to NHS Resolution data?

ANSWER: Anticoagulants, opioids, antimicrobials, antidepressants, anticonvulsants

Test Your Knowledge

1   **What is NHS Resolution?**
    ANSWER: Operating name of NHS Litigation Authority.

2   **What is another name for Human Factors?**
    ANSWER: Ergonomics

3   **What is the estimated number of adverse events per year in NHS England?**
    ANSWER: 850 000

4   **How many of these adverse events are estimated to have been preventable?**
    ANSWER: Half of these = 425,000

5   **What is the overall aim of Human Factors?**
    ANSWER: To minimise errors

6   **What is said to be the focus of Human Factors?**
    ANSWER: Improving efficiency, Job satisfaction and patient safety.

7   **What are the 10 main applications where Human Factors have been incorporated in healthcare?**
    ANSWER: To support teamwork, in healthcare facility design, in re-organising healthcare services, in allocating staffing and resources, in selection and recruitment, in simulation, in technology and device design, to support boards to lead, in investigation and learning, in developing safe protocols and procedures

8   **What is the number of claims reviewed by NHS Resolution for drug administration errors from 1/4/2015–31/3/2020?**
    ANSWER: 146 claims reviewed

CHAPTER 3

Activity 3.1

What does the ERA in the ERA cycle of reflection stand for?
ANSWER: E = Experience, R = Reflection, A = Action

Test Your Knowledge

Think of an incident in your working life, and document it using the Rolf et al Model of Reflection.
ANSWER: How many of you checked for the answer? D'oh! Sorry, I don't know the incident you wrote about, but good that you have reflected on your experience using this model.

CHAPTER 4

Test Your Knowledge

You may be a student nurse, a midwife, a nurse associate, or even a newly qualified nurse or overseas nurse, but you will need to revalidate with the NMC after qualification. So, it is important that you have an understanding of the revalidation process. What are the NMC revalidation requirements?

165

ANSWER:

Documentation	Requirements
Practice hours	Minimum practice hours required for a nurse, midwife, nursing associate, nurse and specialist community public health nurse (SCPHN), midwife, and SCPHN = 450 hours. Or 900 hours if renewing two registrations, e.g. both nurse and midwife. Or 1350 hours if renewing three registration, e.g. nurse, midwife, and nursing associate
Continuing professional development	35 hours of continuing professional development (CPD) in the 3-year period since the last renewal or since the individual joined the register. Of the 35 hours, at least 20 hours must have included participatory learning.
Practice-related feedback	This can be verbal, formal, or informal and come from patients and service users, colleagues, or management. This feedback can also come from team performance reports or annual appraisals. This feedback needs to be documented.
Written reflective account	5 written reflective accounts in the 3-year period since the last renewal or since the individual joined the register.
Reflective discussion	Reflective discussion with another NMC registrant covering the 5 written reflective accounts on the individual's CPD and/or practice-related feedback and/or an event or experience in the individual's practice and how this relates to the code.
Health and character	A declaration of health and character must be provided – fitness to practice.
Professional indemnity arrangement	Most employers provide an indemnity arrangement – individuals will need to check this. Self-employed individuals will need to arrange their own professional indemnity cover.
Confirmation	A confirmer will need to declare that the individual has met the revalidation requirement.

CHAPTER 5

Activity 5.1

Think of an incident in your work environment, and try some free writing to de-clutter the incident from your mind. Remember, no one needs to see this writing unless you want them to.
ANSWER: How many of you checked for the answer? D'oh! Sorry, I don't know the incident you wrote about, but good that you have reflected on your experience using this form of writing.

Activity 5.2

How not to write reflectively: Elliot works in a residential care home and wrote his reflective piece using **text talk** when using the Rolf et al. Model of Reflection. What the heck does it all mean?

What?	I did not check SU BG B4 admin. Insulin 😕
So what?	AFAIK this can be srsly dangerous if SU's BG is very low & NSFL. FYI instead of insulin, in this 💼 they require glucose 🥤 ASAP
Now what?	Ngl, TIL I need 2 follow CH protocol. I will always check BG from now on 😊

ANSWER:

What?	I did not check the Service User's blood glucose before administering insulin.
So what?	As far as I know, this can be seriously dangerous if the Service User's blood glucose is very low and not safe for life. For your information, instead of insulin, in this case they require glucose snacks and drinks as soon as possible.
Now what?	Not gonna lie, today I learned I need to follow the Care Homes protocol. I will always check blood glucose from now on.

Test Your Knowledge

Think of an incident in your working life, and document it using Kolb's Experiential Learning Cycle Model of Reflection.
ANSWER: How many of you checked for the answer? D'oh! Sorry, I don't know the incident you wrote about, but good that you have reflected on your experience using this model.

CHAPTER 6

Activity 6.1

Think back to Chapter 5. What are the important features of reflective writing?
ANSWER:
- Is written in a personal manner – Using personal pronouns, such as 'I', 'me', and 'my'

- Investigates an experience in a focused manner – Using only one or two topics
- Critically analyses what has happened – Using relevant literature to link experience to theory
- Highlights implications for the future – Applying what you have learned to your future practice.

Test Your Knowledge

Think of the last learning event you attended, and reflect on it using the NMC Reflective Account questions:

1 **What was the nature of the CPD activity and/or practice-related feedback and/or event or experience in your practice?**

2 **What did you learn from the CPD activity and/or feedback and/or event or experience in your practice?**

3 **How did you change or improve your practice as a result?**

4 **How is this relevant to the Code?**
ANSWER: This is personal to you.

CHAPTER 7

Activity 7.1

Can critical incident analysis be applied to both positive and negative situations?
ANSWER: Yes.

Test Your Knowledge

Think of an incident in your working life, and document it using the Weather Model of reflection.
ANSWER: How many of you checked for the answer! D'oh! Sorry, but I don't know the incident that you wrote about, but good that you have reflected on your experience using this model.

CHAPTER 8

Test Your Knowledge

1 What are the traits of a 'grand plan' writer?
ANSWER: The grand plan writer reads and makes notes and leaves writing a plan or beginning the writing process until they have an almost complete picture of the essay ready in their head.

2 What are the percentages of the process of preparing, thinking, and planning for an assignment?
ANSWER: 9%

3 What are the components of the CRAAP literature search?
ANSWER:
Currency: When was the information created?
Relevance: Is the information related to our search?
Accuracy: Is the information factual?

Authority: Who created the information? Has it been peer reviewed?
Purpose: Why was the information created (to inform, teach, sell, etc.)?

4 What does the process word 'analyse' mean?
ANSWER: Identify the main points and significant features. Examine critically and/or in great detail.

5 What does the process word 'compare' mean?
ANSWER: Show similarities between two (or more) things. Indicate relevance, importance, and consequence of these similarities.

6 What does the process word 'contrast' mean?
ANSWER: Show differences between two (or more) things. Indicate relevance, importance, and consequence of these differences. If appropriate, justify why one item/ argument may be more convincing or preferred.

7 What does the process word 'criticise' mean?
ANSWER: Make a judgement – based on and using examples, evidence, and reasoning – about

the merit of two or more related things: for example, theories, opinions, models, items.

8 What does the process word 'critically evaluate' mean?
ANSWER: Weigh arguments for and against something, indicating and then assessing the strength of the evidence on both sides. Be clear about your criteria for how you judge which side is preferable/more convincing.

9 What does the process word 'reflect' mean?
ANSWER: Think deeply or carefully about.

10 What does the process word 'synthesis' mean?
ANSWER: Combine information and ideas from multiple sources to develop and strengthen the argument (s)

Chapter 9	Put your feet up.
Chapter 10	Have a biscuit and a
Chapter 11	cup of tea or coffee –
Chapter 12	nothing for you to
Chapter 13	do now, apart from
Chapter 14	reading through the
Chapter 15	reflective accounts.

Index

Reflective Practice for Nurses, First Edition. Claire Boyd.
© 2023 John Wiley & Sons Ltd. Published 2023 by John Wiley & Sons Ltd.